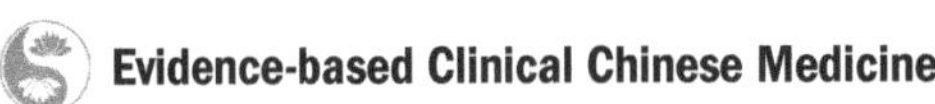 Evidence-based Clinical Chinese Medicine

Volume 10

Diabetic Kidney Disease

Evidence-based Clinical Chinese Medicine

Print ISSN: 2529-7562
Online ISSN: 2529-7554

Series Co Editors-in-Chief

Charlie Changli Xue *(RMIT University, Australia)*
Chuanjian Lu *(Guangdong Provincial Hospital of Chinese Medicine, China)*

Published

Forthcoming

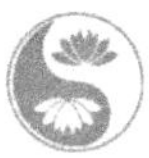 **Evidence-based Clinical Chinese Medicine**

Co Editors-in-Chief

Charlie Changli Xue
RMIT University, Australia

Chuanjian Lu
Guangdong Provincial Hospital of Chinese Medicine, China

Volume 10
Diabetic Kidney Disease

Lead Authors

Johannah Shergis
RMIT University, Australia

Lihong Yang
Guangdong Provincial Hospital of Chinese Medicine, China

World Scientific

NEW JERSEY · LONDON · SINGAPORE · BEIJING · SHANGHAI · HONG KONG · TAIPEI · CHENNAI · TOKYO

Published by

World Scientific Publishing Co. Pte. Ltd.

5 Toh Tuck Link, Singapore 596224

USA office: 27 Warren Street, Suite 401-402, Hackensack, NJ 07601

UK office: 57 Shelton Street, Covent Garden, London WC2H 9HE

Library of Congress Cataloging-in-Publication Data
Names: Xue, Charlie Changli, author. | Lu, Chuan-jian, 1964–   author.
Title: Evidence-based clinical Chinese medicine / Charlie Changli Xue, Chuanjian Lu.
Description: New Jersey : World Scientific, 2016. | Includes bibliographical references and index.
Identifiers: LCCN 2015030389| ISBN 9789814723084 (v. 1 : hardcover : alk. paper) |
   ISBN 9789814723091 (v. 1 : paperback : alk. paper) |
   ISBN 9789814723121 (v. 2 : hardcover : alk. paper) |
   ISBN 9789814723138 (v. 2 : paperback : alk. paper) |
   ISBN 9789814759045 (v. 3 : hardcover : alk. paper) |
   ISBN 9789814759052 (v. 3 : paperback : alk. paper)
Subjects: | MESH: Medicine, Chinese Traditional--methods. | Clinical Medicine--methods. |
   Evidence-Based Medicine--methods. | Psoriasis. | Pulmonary Disease, Chronic Obstructive.
Classification: LCC RC81 | NLM WB 55.C4 | DDC 616--dc23
LC record available at http://lccn.loc.gov/2015030389

Volume 10: Diabetic Kidney Disease
ISBN 978-981-3276-10-9 (hardcover)
ISBN 978-981-123-535-1 (paperback)
ISBN 978-981-3276-11-6 (ebook for institutions)
ISBN 978-981-3276-12-3 (ebook for individuals)

First published 2019
Reprinted 2021

British Library Cataloguing-in-Publication Data
A catalogue record for this book is available from the British Library.

For any available supplementary material, please visit
https://www.worldscientific.com/worldscibooks/10.1142/11151#t=suppl

Disclaimer

The information in this monograph is based on systematic analyses of the best available evidence for Chinese medicine interventions both historical and contemporary. Every effort has been made to ensure accuracy and completeness of the data of this publication. This book is intended for clinicians, researchers and educators. The practice of evidence-based medicine consists of consideration of the best available evidence, practitioners' clinical experience and judgment, and patients' preference. Not all interventions are acceptable in all countries. It is important to note that some of the substances mentioned in this book may no longer be in use, may be toxic, or be prohibited or restricted under the provisions of the Convention on International Trade in Endangered Species of Wild Fauna and Flora (CITES). Practitioners, researchers and educators are advised to comply with the relevant regulations in their country and with the restrictions on the trade in species included in CITES appendices I, II and III. This book is not intended as a guide for self-medication. Patients should seek professional advice from qualified Chinese medicine practitioners.

Foreword

Since the late 20th century, Chinese medicine, including acupuncture and herbal medicine, has been increasingly used throughout the world. The parallel development and spread of evidence-based medicine has provided challenges and opportunities for Chinese medicine.

The opportunities have been evidence-based medicine's emphasis on the effective use of the best available clinical evidence, incorporating the clinicians' clinical experience, subject to patients' preference. Such practices have a patient focus which reflects the historical nature of Chinese medicine practice. However, the challenges are also significant due to the fact that, despite the long term development and very rich literature accumulated over 2,000 years, there is an overall lack of high level clinical evidence for many of the interventions used in Chinese medicine.

To address this knowledge gap, we need to generate clinical evidence through high quality clinical studies and to evaluate evidence to enable effective use of such available evidence to promote evidence-based Chinese medicine practice.

Modern Chinese medicine is rooted in its classical literature and the legacies of ancient doctors, grounded in the practice of expert clinicians and increasingly informed by clinical and experimental research efforts. In recognition of the unique features of Chinese medicine, for each of the conditions in this series a 'Whole Evidence' approach is used to provide a synthesis of different types and levels of evidence to enable practitioners to make clinical decisions informed by the current best evidence.

There are four main components of this 'Whole Evidence' approach. First, we present the current approaches to the diagnosis, differentiation and treatment of each condition based on expert consensus in published textbooks and clinical guidelines. This provides an overview of how the condition is currently managed. The second section provides an analysis of the condition in historical context based on systematic searches of the *Zhong Hua Yi Dian* which includes the full texts of more than 1,000 classical medical books. These analyses provide objective views on how the condition has been treated over two millennia, reveal continuities and discontinuities between traditional and modern practice, and suggest avenues for future research.

The third component is the assessment of evidence derived from modern clinical studies of Chinese medicine interventions. The methods established by the *Cochrane Collaboration* are used as the basis for conducting systematic reviews and undertaking meta-analyses of outcome data for randomised controlled trials (RCTs). In addition, the clinical relevance of meta-analysis data is enhanced by examining the herbal formulae, individual herbs and acupuncture treatments that were assessed in the RCTs and the evidence base is broadened by the inclusion of data from controlled clinical trials and non-controlled studies. The fourth component is to determine how the herbal medicine interventions may achieve the effects indicated by the clinical trials. Thus for each of the most frequently used herbs we provide reviews of their effects in pre-clinical models and their likely mechanisms of action.

For each condition, this 'Whole Evidence' approach links clinical expertise, historical precedent, clinical research data and experimental research to provide the reader with assessments of the current state of the evidence of efficacy and safety for Chinese medicine interventions using herbal medicines, acupuncture and moxibustion and other health care practices such as *tai chi*.

Since these books are available in Chinese and English, they can benefit patients, practitioners and educators internationally and enable practitioners to make clinical decisions informed by the current best evidence.

These publications represent a major milestone in Chinese medicine development and make a significant contribution to the evidence-based Chinese medicine development globally.

Co-Editors-in-Chief

Professor Charlie Changli Xue, RMIT University, Australia

Professor Chuanjian Lu, Guangdong Provincial Hospital of Chinese Medicine, China

Purpose of the Monograph

This book is intended for clinicians, researchers and educators. It can be used to inform tertiary education and clinical practice by providing systematic, multi-dimensional assessments of the best available evidence for using Chinese medicine to manage each common clinical condition.

How to Use this Monograph

Some Definitions

A glossary is included, containing terms and definitions which frequently appear in the book. It also describes the definitions of statistical tests, methodological terms, evaluation tools and interventions. For example, in this book, Integrative Medicine refers to the combined use of a Chinese medicine treatment with conventional medical management, and Combination Therapies refers to two or more Chinese medicines from different therapy groups (Chinese herbal medicine, acupuncture or other Chinese medicine therapies) administered together. Terminology used throughout the monograph is based on the World Health Organisation's *Standard Terminologies on Traditional Medicine in the Western Pacific Region* (2007) where possible or from the cited reference.

Data Analysis and Interpretation of Results

In order to synthesise the clinical evidence, a range of statistical analysis approaches are used. In general, the effect size for dichotomous data is reported as a risk ratio (RR) with 95% confidence intervals (CI), and for continuous data, they are reported as mean difference (MD) with 95% CI. Statistically significant effects are indicated with an asterisk*. Readers should note that statistical significant does not necessarily correspond with a clinically important effect. Interpretation of results should take into consideration of the clinical significance, quality of studies (expressed as high, low or unclear risk of bias in this book) and heterogeneity amongst the studies. Tests for heterogeneity are conducted using the I^2 statistic. An I^2 score greater than 50% may indicate substantial heterogeneity.

Use of Evidence in Practice

The Grading of Recommendations Assessment, Development and Evaluation (GRADE) approach was used to summarise the quality of evidence and results of the strength of evidence for critical and important comparisons and outcomes. Due to the diverse nature of Chinese medicine practice, treatment recommendations are not included with the summary of findings tables. Therefore readers will need to interpret the evidence with reference to the local practice environment.

Limitations

Readers should note some of the methodological limitations on classical literature and clinical evidence.

- Search terms used to search the *Zhong Hua Yi Dian* database may not include all terms that have been used for the condition, which may alter the findings.
- Chinese language has changed over time. Citations have been interpreted for analysis, and such interpretations may be subject to disagreement.
- Chinese medicine theory has evolved over time. As such, concepts described in classical Chinese medical literature may no longer be found in contemporary works.

- Symptoms described in citations may be common to many conditions, and a judgment was required to determine the likelihood of the citation being related to the condition. This may have introduced some bias due to the subjective nature of the judgment.
- The vast majority of the clinical evidence for Chinese medicine treatments has come from China. The applicability of the findings to other populations and other countries requires further assessment.
- Many studies included participants with varying disease severity. Where possible, subgroup analyses were undertaken to examine the effects in different sub-populations. As this was not always possible, the findings may be limited to the population included, and not to sub-populations.
- The potential risk of bias found in many included studies suggested methodological limitations. The findings for GRADE assessments based on studies of very low to moderate quality evidence should be interpreted accordingly.
- Nine major English and Chinese language databases were searched to identify clinical studies, in addition to clinical trial registers. Other studies may exist which were not identified through searches, and which may alter the findings.
- The calculation of frequency of herbal formula use was based on formula names only. It is possible that studies evaluated herbal treatments with the same or similar herb ingredients, but which were given different formula names. Due to the complexity of herbal formulas, it was considered not appropriate to make a judgment as to the similarity of formulas for analysis. As such, the frequency of formulas reported in Chapter 5 may be underestimated.
- The most frequently utilised herbs which may have contributed to the treatment effect have been described in Chapter 5. These herbs may provide leads for further exploration. Calculation of the herbs with potential effect is based on frequency of formulae reported in the studies, and doesn't take into consideration the clinical implications and functions of every herb in a formula.

Authors and Contributors

Co-Editors-in-Chief

Prof. Charlie Changli Xue (*RMIT University, Australia*)
Prof. Chuanjian Lu (*Guangdong Provincial Hospital of Chinese Medicine, China*)

Co-Deputy Editors-in-Chief

Assoc. Prof. Anthony Lin Zhang (*RMIT University, Australia*)
Dr. Brian H May (*RMIT University, Australia*)
Prof. Xinfeng Guo (*Guangdong Provincial Hospital of Chinese Medicine, China*)
Prof. Zehuai Wen (*Guangdong Provincial Hospital of Chinese Medicine, China*)

Lead Authors

Dr. Johannah Shergis (*RMIT University, Australia*)
Dr. Lihong Yang (*Guangdong Provincial Hospital of Chinese Medicine, China*)

Co-Authors

RMIT University (Australia):
Assoc. Prof. Anthony Lin Zhang
Prof. Charlie Changli Xue

Guangdong Provincial Hospital of Chinese Medicine (China):

Prof. Chuanjian Lu
Dr. La Zhang
Dr. Lei Zhang
Prof. Xinfeng Guo
Prof. Xusheng Liu
Prof. Zehuai Wen

Members of Advisory Committee and Panel

Prof. Peter J Coloe (*RMIT University, Australia*)
Prof. Yubo Lyu (*Guangdong Provincial Hospital of Chinese Medicine, China*)
Prof. Dacan Chen (*Guangdong Provincial Hospital of Chinese Medicine, China*)

Prof. Keji Chen (*The Chinese Academy of Sciences, China*)
Prof. Aiping Lu (*Hong Kong Baptist University, China*)
Prof. Caroline Smith (*University of Western Sydney, Australia*)
Prof. David F Story (*RMIT University, Australia*)

Prof. Zhaoxiang Bian (*Hong Kong Baptist University, China*)
The Late Prof. George Lewith (*University of Southampton, United Kingdom*)
Prof. Jianping Liu (*Beijing University of Chinese Medicine, China*)
Prof. Frank Thien (*Monash University, Australia*)
Prof. Jialiang Wang (*Sichuan University, China*)
Prof. Lixing Lao (*The University of Hong Kong, China*)

Prof. Wei Mao (*Guangdong Provincial Hospital of Chinese Medicine, China*)

Prof. David Johnson (*Australasian Kidney Trials Network, University of Queensland, Princess Alexandra Hospital, Translational Research Institute, Australia*)
Prof. Jian min Li (*Beijing Hospital of Integrated Traditional Chinese and Western Medicine, China*)
Prof. Ying Lu (*Tongde Hospital of Zhejiang Province, China*)
Dr. George Wu (*Credit Valley Hospital, Canada*)

Professor Charlie Changli Xue, PhD

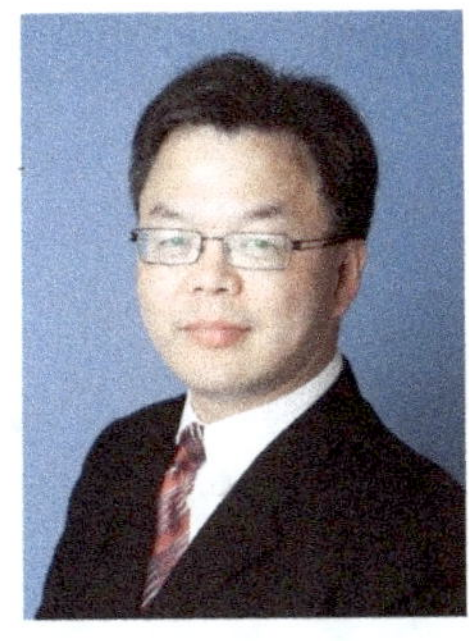

Professor Charlie Changli Xue holds a Bachelor of Medicine (majoring in Chinese Medicine) from Guangzhou University of Chinese Medicine, China (1987) and a PhD from RMIT University, Australia (2000). He has been an academic, researcher, regulator and practitioner for almost three decades. Professor Xue has made significant contributions to evidence-based educational development, clinical research, regulatory framework and policy development and provision of high quality clinical care to the community. Professor Xue is recognised internationally as an expert in evidence-based traditional medicine and integrative healthcare.

Professor Xue is the Inaugural National Chair of the Chinese Medicine Board of Australia appointed by the Australian Health Workforce Ministerial Council (in 2011), and he was reappointed for the second term in 2014. Since 2007, he has been a Member of the World Health Organization (WHO) Expert Advisory Panel for Traditional and Complementary Medicine, Geneva. Professor Xue is also Honorary Senior Principal Research Fellow at the Guangdong Provincial Academy of Chinese Medical Sciences, China.

At RMIT, Professor Xue is Executive Dean, School of Health and Biomedical Sciences. He is also Director, World Health Organization (WHO) Collaborating Centre for Traditional Medicine.

Between 1995 and 2010, Professor Xue was Discipline Head of Chinese Medicine at RMIT University. He leads the development of five successful undergraduate and postgraduate degree programs in

Chinese Medicine at RMIT University which is now a global leader in Chinese medicine education and research.

Professor Xue's research has been supported by over AU$15 million research grants including six project grants from the Australian Government's National Health & Medical Research Council (NHMRC) and two Australian Research Council (ARC) grants. He has contributed over 200 publications and has been frequently invited as keynote speaker for numerous national and international conferences. Professor Xue has contributed to over 300 media interviews on issues related to complementary medicine education, research, regulation and practice.

Professor Chuanjian Lu, MD

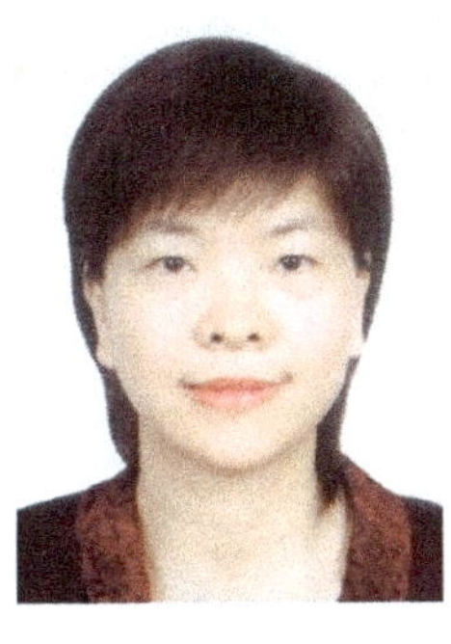

Professor Chuanjian Lu, Doctor of Medicine. She is the vice president of Guangdong Provincial Hospital of Chinese Medicine (Guangdong Provincial Academy of Chinese Medical Sciences, Second Clinical Medical College of Guangzhou University of Chinese Medicine). She also is the chair of the Guangdong Traditional Chinese Medicine (TCM) Standardization Technical Committee, and the vice-chair of the Immunity Specialty Committee of the World Federation of Chinese Medicine Societies (WFCMS).

Professor Lu has engaged in scientific research into TCM, clinical practice and teaching for some 25 years. Her research has been devoted to integrated traditional and western medicine. She has edited and published 12 monographs and 120 academic research articles as first author and corresponding author with over 30 articles being included in SCI journals.

She has received widespread recognition for her achievements with awards for "Excellent Teacher of South China", "National Outstanding Women TCM Doctor", and "National Outstanding Young Doctor of TCM". She also received "The Science and Technology Star of the Association of Chinese Medicine", the "National Excellent Science and Technology Workers of China Award" and the "Five-Continent Women's Scientific Awards of China Medical Women's Association".

Professor Lu has won the Award of Science and Technology Progress over 10 times from Guangdong Provincial Government, China Association of Chinese Medicine and Chinese Hospital Association.

Acknowledgements

The authors and contributors would like to acknowledge the valuable contributions of the following people who assisted with database searches, data extraction, data screening, data assessment, translation of documents, editing, and/or administrative tasks: Mr Jianlin Jian, Mr Chunpeng Wang, Mr Kai Zhou, Mr Guirui Huang, Ms Jialing Liu, Ms Jueyao Liang and Ms Jiaqi Lai. We also acknowledge the assistance of Dr Neil Owens in editing the monograph.

Contents

Contents

List of Figures

List of Tables

1

Introduction to Diabetic Kidney Disease

OVERVIEW

Diabetic kidney disease (DKD) is caused by diabetes mellitus. Over time, high levels of blood glucose damage the kidney's filtering system, leading to kidney impairment and eventually failure. DKD affects millions of people globally and its impact is still ever increasing due to an ageing population and growing prevalence of diabetes. People with diabetes may not know they have DKD because in the early stages it is asymptomatic. Effective treatments targeting renal damage are limited. The mainstay of therapy is controlling blood glucose levels and reducing high blood pressure. This chapter describes the definition, risk factors, epidemiological profile, pathological processes, diagnosis and treatment of DKD.

Definition of Diabetic Kidney Disease

Clinical Presentation of Diabetic Kidney Disease

Diabetic kidney disease (DKD), previously known as diabetic nephropathy is a clinical syndrome characterised by persistent albuminuria and progressive loss of kidney function caused by diabetes mellitus (DM).[1] It is the foremost microvascular complication of DM and more often develops in those with chronically poor glycaemic control.[2]

DKD can develop from all types of diabetes, including Type 1 (insulin dependent) and Type 2 (non-insulin dependent) diabetes. It may be asymptomatic in the early stages, or symptoms may include oedema, breathlessness when lying flat (orthopnoea) due to pulmonary oedema, and altered urine due to proteinuria. In advanced DKD, hypertension, increased oedema, or symptoms of other diabetic complications, such as blurry vision and numbness in the extremities can be found.[1] For patients that develop advanced DKD, symptoms of uraemia may be the chief complaint.

Epidemiology

As the hallmark of DKD, albuminuria or impaired glomerular filtration rate (GFR) is observed in around 25–53% of diabetes patients.[3-5] The number of people with diabetes has been rising for decades. The International Diabetes Federation estimates that the number of people with diabetes will rise from 415 million (8.8%) of the global population aged 20–79 years old in 2015 to 642 million (10.4%) by 2040.[6] Thus, the number of people with DKD is very likely to be continually growing in the future.[6,7] The prevalence of DKD in people with diabetes from each continent is presented in Table 1.1.

Table 1.1.   Prevalence of Diabetic Kidney Disease in People with Diabetes

Continents	Prevalence of DKD based on Diabetic Populations
North America	30.9%–34.5%[3,8]
Asia	26.1%–52.5%[4,9,10]
Africa	9.8%–50%[11]
Europe	25.6%–51%[7,12]
Australia	25.1%[5]

Burden

The direct and indirect costs of DKD are high, mostly due to cardiovascular complications and the development of end stage renal disease (ESRD). DKD accounts for approximately 50% of new dialysis patients in the United States and 30% in Australia.[13,14] In addition, DKD patients have a higher risk of cardiovascular morbidity and mortality than those with diabetes or chronic kidney disease (CKD) alone.[15] The age standardised death rate of CKD due to diabetes rose from 1.4% per 100,000 population in 1990 to 2.9% in 2013.[16] Each year in Australia, approximately 3,000 deaths are caused by diabetes in association with kidney failure.[17]

In the US, medical costs for patients with CKD and diabetes rose 70.2% between 2008 and 2012, nearly $25,000 per patient-year, while similar costs for patients without CKD, diabetes, or chronic heart failure increased by only 4.1%.[13] In Australia, DKD accounts for a substantial economic burden. The total direct health care costs reached almost $1 billion per annum for early stage DKD and $300 million for ESRD patients.[5] As the number of people with diabetes increases, demands for disease screening and renal therapies will continually grow, resulting in a heavy health care burden.

Risk Factors

The pathogenesis of DKD is complex and includes genetic as well as environmental factors. Risk factors are either modifiable or irreversible. Modifiable risk factors may include poor glycaemic control, hypertension, obesity and smoking.[18-20] The progression of DKD often relates to the degree of hyperglycaemic control and duration of diabetes.

Irreversible risk factors include a family history of diabetes, predisposing genes, ethnicity, male gender, and advanced age.[21-23] Though familial DKD is frequently observed, identification of causative genes is difficult. Among the candidate genes, genetic polymorphisms of methylenetetrahydrofolate reductase, angiotensin converting enzyme (ACE) genes and aldose reductase were found to be related to the initiation of DKD.[24,25] In addition, Mexican-Americans, African-Americans, and Pima Indians are at higher risk of DKD.[26-28] Despite these known risk factors, none are predictive of DKD onset or progression in an individual patient.

Pathological Processes

The pathogenesis of DKD is not fully understood. However, studies suggest it is initiated by activation of metabolic, inflammatory and

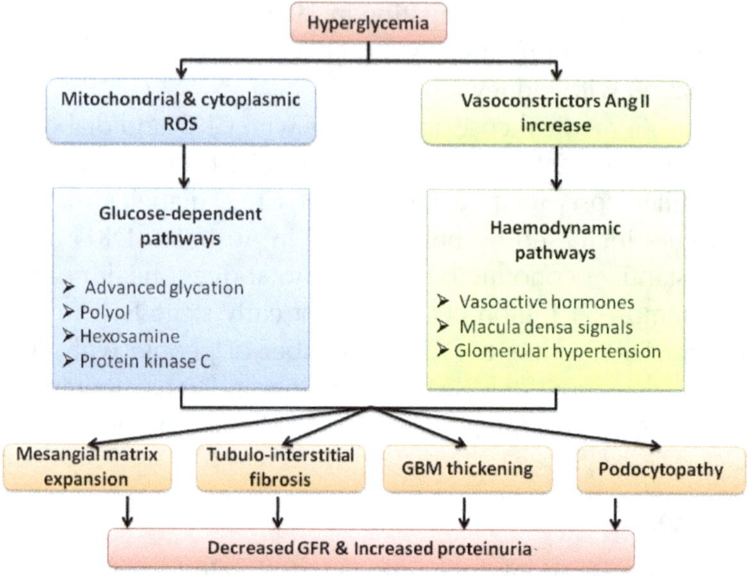

Fig. 1.1. Pathological process of diabetic kidney disease

Abbreviations: Ang II, angiotensin II; GBM, glomerular basement membrane; GFR, glomerular hypertension rate; ROS, reactive oxygen species.

hemodynamic pathways.[29] These three main pathways overlap and can influence each other (Fig. 1.1).

Long-term hyperglycaemia is pivotal in the development of DKD. This leads to increased protein kinase C activity, excess profibrotic cytokines and growth factor secretion, abnormal polyol metabolism, glycosylation of renal proteins and generation of advanced glycation end products (AGEs).[30] Accumulated pathological products generated from the above pathways also induce expression of reactive oxygen species (ROS), causing free radical injury and, along with inflammatory processes, acceleration of the development of DKD.[31,32]

In addition, haemodynamic disturbances followed by hyperglycaemia increase activity of vasoactive systems, including the renin-angiotensin system (RAS) and endothelin system. Consequently, glomerular afferent arterioles dilate while efferent arterioles constrict, resulting in systemic and intraglomerular hypertension. The hemodynamic change also triggers autocrine and paracrine release of cytokines and growth factors in the glomerulus.[33]

Abnormal metabolic, hemodynamic and inflammatory processes eventually lead to functional and structural changes in the kidneys. Mesangial cells increase in both number and size, associated with extracellular matrix deposition and mesangial expansion. The ensuing mesangial collagen and fibrin deposition and glomerular vascular endothelial damage result in glomerular ischemia and then atrophy, manifesting as nodular lesions under light microscopy. Fibrosis in the tubulointerstitium is caused by increased fibrogenic cytokines, growth factors and local inflammation. Podocyte loss and impaired tubular albumin uptake are also observed.[18] Renal biopsy often shows structural changes in the kidneys of people with DKD before clinical manifestations, such as albuminuria and decreased GFR.

Typical histological changes in the glomeruli of DKD patients include mesangial expansion, glomerular basement membrane (GBM) thickening and glomerular sclerosis.[34,35] Damage to the basement membrane leads to loss of structural integrity of the filtering system leading to protein leakage out into the ultrafiltrate. In some cases, the glomerular sclerosis may manifest as the characteristic nodular appearance named "Kimmelstiel-Wilson lesions".[36] In order to discriminate lesions of various severity, the America Renal Pathology Society developed a pathology classification for DKD in 2010, in which glomerular lesions were defined and the severities of interstitial and vascular lesions were scored (Table 1.2 and 1.3).[37]

Diagnosis

People with DKD may be asymptomatic without any evidence of nephropathy in the early stages. In most patients with diabetes, particularly accompanied with diabetic retinopathy, which indicates microvascular disease, a diagnosis of DKD is considered if there is albuminuria. In later stages of DKD, physical examination may reveal hypertension, oedema, or diabetic complications including numbness or pain at the toes or fingers, hearing and vision impairment, etc.[38]

Table1.2.   Glomerular Pathology Classification of Diabetic Kidney Disease

Class	Description	Inclusion Criteria
I	Mild or nonspecific light microscopy changes and electron microscopy-proven glomerular basement membrane (GBM) thickening	GBM >395 nm in female and >430 nm in male individuals nine years of age and older
IIa	Mild mesangial expansion	Mild mesangial expansion in >25% of the observed mesangium
IIb	Severe mesangial expansion	Severe mesangial expansion in >25% of the observed mesangium
III	Nodular sclerosis (Kimmelstiel-Wilson lesion)	At least one convincing Kimmelstiel-Wilson lesion
IV	Advanced diabetic glomerulosclerosis	Global glomerular sclerosis in >50% of glomeruli; Lesions from classes I through III

Table reference[37]

Table 1.3.   Interstitial and Vascular Lesions of Diabetic Kidney Disease

Lesion	Criteria	Score
Interstitial Lesions		
Interstitial Fibrosis and Tubular Atrophy (IFTA)	No IFTA	0
	<25%	1
	25%–50%	2
	>50%	3
Interstitial Inflammation	Absent	0
	Infiltration only in relation to IFTA	1
	Infiltration in areas without IFTA	2
Vascular Lesions		
Arteriolar hyalinosis	Absent	0
	At least one area of arteriolar hyalinosis	1
	More than one area of arteriolar hyalinosis	2
Presence of large vessels		yes/no
Arteriosclerosis (score worst artery)	No intimal thickening	0
	Intimal thickening less than thickness of media	1
	Intimal thickening greater than thickness of media	2

Table reference[37]

When patients progress to ESRD, symptoms of uraemia, including lethargy, anorexia, nausea and vomiting, may be the chief complaint.

Albuminuria is an early indicator of DKD which was listed as a diagnostic criterion in the early clinical practice guidelines. However, the diagnosis of DKD is not internationally standardised. The Kidney Disease Outcomes Quality Initiative (KDOQI) guideline[39] provides one example of DKD diagnosis and states that abnormalities in albuminuria excretion are categorised as microalbuminuria and macroalbuminuria. In individuals with diabetes showing microalbuminuria or macroalbuminuria plus diabetic retinopathy, it indicates a probable diagnose of DKD. In addition, individuals with type 1 diabetes for at least 10 years who present with microalbuminuria are considered to have DKD.[39]

Albuminuria can be measured differently including a urine spot test for urinary albumin-creatinine ratio (ACR) or urinary timed test for urinary albuminuria excretion rate (AER). Infections, fever, recent vigorous exercise and other factors could falsely elevate albumin excretion and need to be differentiated.

Albuminuria levels are categorised as normal urinary albumin excretion or increased urinary albumin excretion (Table 1.4). The terms microalbuminuria and macroalbuminuria are widely used but are no longer recommended by the American Diabetes Association because of the continuum of albuminuria measurements.[2]

Along with quantitative urinary albumin assessment, serum creatinine should be measured to estimate the GFR. Although albuminuria was an early indicator of DKD, studies have found an

Table 1.4.   Albumin Excretion

Category	Spot Collection (mg/g creatinine)
Normal	<30
Increased urinary albumin excretion	≥30
Microalbuminuria (Moderately increased albuminuria)	30~300
Macroalbuminuria (Severely increased albuminuria)	>300

Table reference[2,39]

increasing proportion (up to 1/3) of type 2 diabetes patients with decreased estimated GFR without increased urinary albumin excretion.[40-42] Therefore diabetes patients with declining GFR, especially those accompanied with diabetic retinopathy, after excluding other underlying causes of kidney disease, would be considered to have impaired kidney function due to DKD.[43]

Since the number of people with diabetes is large and albuminuria can be seen in several conditions, other underlying causes of kidney diseases in diabetic patients should be taken into considered when making a diagnosis. The 2007 KDOQI guidelines recommend considering non-diabetic causes if there is[39]:

- Absence of diabetic retinopathy;
- Low or rapidly decreasing GFR;
- Rapidly increasing proteinuria or presence of nephrotic syndrome;
- Refractory hypertension;
- Presence of active urinary sediment;
- Signs or symptoms of other systemic disease; or
- >30% reduction in GFR within 2–3 months after initiation of angiotensin-converting enzyme inhibitors (ACEi) or angiotensin II receptor blockers (ARB) medications.

In patients with unclear aetiology or when other causes of kidney disease are suspected, renal biopsy can be performed to definitively diagnose diabetic glomerulopathy. However, in patients with type 2 diabetes and microalbuminuria, 30% of them may have normal or near normal biopsy results.[44] In order to distinguish nephropathies from other underlying causes in the diabetic population, the term DKD, instead of diabetic nephropathy is applied as a presumptive diagnosis of kidney disease caused by diabetes. Meanwhile, the term diabetic glomerulopathy is reserved for biopsy-proven kidney injury caused by diabetes.[39]

Management

The medical management of DKD requires a multifaceted and interdisciplinary approach. The main components are management of primary disease, that is diabetes, and the management of risk factors, such as hypertension and dyslipidaemia.[45] Lifestyle adjustment and patient's self-managed education are also important in managing diabetes and DKD.

Non-pharmacological Management

Since lifestyle and diet are closely related to diabetes, instructions about healthy behaviours to reduce risk factors of DKD may have substantial clinical benefits. Smoking cessation, adequate physical activity, and maintaining a normal range of body mass index are essential for both diabetes and DKD. As for diet modification, current guidelines recommend a daily protein intake of 0.8 g/kg body weight for non-dialysis DKD patients and higher protein intake for dialysis patients.[2,39] Low-protein diets (daily intake <0.8 g/kg body weight) are not recommended because they do not alter glycaemic measures or slow GFR decline.[2]

Pharmacological Management

Treatments for DKD include those that target the primary disease, diabetes as well as treatments that reduce renal damage. Treatments include glycaemic control, antihypertensive therapy, and lipid lowering therapy.

Glycaemic control

As a trigger and progressive factor, glycaemic control is central to the prevention and management of DKD. Strict glycaemic control by maintaining hemoglobinA1c (HbA1c) at around 7% not only reduces the risk of developing microalbuminuria but also reduces long-term risk of impaired GFR.[46–48]

Benefits of strict glycaemic control for prevention of DKD can be observed even after patients return to less intensive glycaemic management. In a recent study, after termination of intense glycaemic control, patients under intense glycaemic control remained at lower risk of microalbuminuria, myocardial infarction and all-cause mortality in the subsequent 10 years.[46,48] The ongoing benefit of strict glycaemic control contributes to the "metabolic memory" effect which highlights the importance of early glycaemic control.[49]

The therapeutic goal of glycaemic control is to maintain HbA1c levels at about 7% to prevent or delay progression of DKD.[50] But this figure may be different in different subgroups of DKD populations.[50] Several large trials showed that tighter glycaemic goal (HbA1c less than 7%) was associated with higher risk of mortality without significant reduction in cardiovascular death.[51,52] Benefit of strict glycaemic control must be counterbalanced by the possible harm of increased hypoglycaemic episodes when planning for optimal glucose control.[2,52]

When selecting glucose lowering medication, renal function, co-morbidity, age, and other risk factors for hypoglycaemia such as severe malnutrition should be taken into consideration, especially in those with advanced DKD. Degradation of some anti-diabetic drugs and their active metabolites are carried out by the kidneys and decreasing clearance caused by impaired kidney function may lead to higher risk of hypoglycaemia and other side effects. Therefore, dosage of glucose lowering medications needs to be evaluated and adjusted based on GFR.[50] Antidiabetic type and dose may vary according to severity or stage of CKD. Treatments may include insulin, meglitinides, biguanides, thiazolidinediones, sulfonylureas, dipeptidyl peptidase-4 (DPP-4) inhibitors, alpha-glucosidase inhibitors, and incretin mimetics.[49,50,54,55]

Blood pressure control

Hypertension is another important independent risk factor for DKD initiation and progression.[56,57] Control of BP is regarded as one of the key strategies to slow down the renal function decline and to reduce risk of mortality in DKD.[53] Anti-hypertensive medications including inhibitors of RAS show additional renal protection properties independent of BP reducing effects.[58-63] For example, a clinical trial found that olmesartan in patients with type 2 diabetes mellitus was associated with a delayed onset of microalbuminuria. The time to the onset of microalbuminuria was increased by 23% in the olmesartan group with a median follow-up of 3.2 years.[64] Therefore, RAS inhibitors, including angiotensin-converting enzyme inhibitors (ACEi) and angiotensin receptor blockers (ARBs), are often used for BP control in patients with DKD. In diabetic patients with albuminuria excretion greater than 30mg/g, ACEi or ARB are also recommended regardless of their hypertension status.[2,50]

The efficacy and safety of dual RAS inhibitors is not clear. Dual therapy of ACEi plus ARB can reduce the risk of ESRD compared with single therapy ARB.[65] However, a recent clinical trial that tested the effect of dual therapy of ACEi with ARB was stopped early due to increased risk of hyperkaelemia and acute kidney injury (AKI), and the trend towards benefit on ESRD was decreased with time.[66] Another study evaluated a combination of half doses of ACEi and ARB compared with single agents at higher doses but did not show benefit in terms of progression and the incidence of adverse events were similar between groups.[67] Current guidelines do not recommend the dual use of RAS inhibitors. Some research suggests that the undesired effects may be caused by inappropriate comparisons and BP targets, inappropriate drug additions, and unclear adverse events criteria.[68–70] Network meta-analysis showed that the estimated risks of hyperkaelemia or AKI of dual therapy were not statistically significant but trended towards increased risks.[65]

Blood pressure should be controlled for non-dialysis DKD patients at less than 130/80 mmHg.[2,50,71] Despite the current evidence the precise BP control still needs further research to better understand the optimal range. In addition, BP targets are hard to achieve and may require combinations of different classes of antihypertensive drugs.

Diuretics and calcium channel blockers can be used in addition to ACEi or ARB to achieve target BP. However, serum creatinine should be monitored when a combination of diuretics and RAS inhibitors are used.[2] Non-dihydropyridine calcium channel blockers may also reduce proteinuria.[72] Their anti-proteinuric effects can be enhanced by sodium restriction when combined with ACEi.[73] Thus non-dihydropyridine calcium channel blockers can replace RAS inhibitors in DKD patients with contraindications or intolerance.

The mineralocorticoid receptor antagonists (MRA), eplerenone and spironolactone, have been shown to reduce proteinuria in DKD patients who are already taking either an ACEi or ARB. However, the anti-proteinuric effect has been offset by a three- to eightfold increased risk of hyperkaelemia. A new nonsteroidal MRA, finerenone, has shown greater receptor selectivity than spironolactone and better receptor affinity than eplerenone in *in vitro* studies.[74] A randomised phase 2 trial found that, compared to placebo, finerenone reduced albuminuria excretion by at least 21% at 90 days against a background of RAS inhibition, while hyperkaelemia occurred at a rate of just 1.5%.[75] Longer-term studies that assess the effect on GFR and albuminuria over time are needed.

Lipid management

It is still unclear if the level of lipids plays a significant role in the pathogenesis of DKD. Although dyslipidaemia is associated with increased albuminuria excretion in diabetes patients,[76–78] there is lack of compelling evidence that lipid lowering therapy affects the rate of CKD (including DKD) progression. Nevertheless, lipid lowering therapy (at least statins) reduced the risks of death, major adverse cardiovascular events (non-fatal myocardial infarction, non-haemorrhagic stroke, or any arterial revascularisation procedure) in CKD patients including those with diabetes.[79,80] Therefore, KDOQI guidelines recommend that use of low-density lipoprotein cholesterol (LDL-C) lowering medication (e.g. statins or statin/ezetimibe combination) to achieve a target of LDL-C less than 100 mg/dL (2.6 mmol/L) for patients with CKD and diabetes.[39,50]

The effects of statins are dose-dependent. Namely, higher doses produce greater benefits. However, it is accompanied by an increased risk of adverse events. Moreover, patients with impaired kidney functions are at high risk of pharmaceutical-related adverse events. Thus dose adjustment is generally needed. Lipid lowering therapy is still recommended in guidelines, but given the potential for toxicity with higher doses of statins and uncertain benefits, target LDL-C was replaced by risk status assessment during the treatment of DKD.[53]

Limitations of Pharmacological Management

Though RAS inhibitors can decrease albuminuria excretion, a network meta-analysis showed that BP lowering agents were not more effective than placebo in prolonging survival in DKD patients.[65] Similarly, persistent loss of renal function occurs in some DKD patients even if current treatment targets are achieved.[81,82] Therefore, despite the treatment modalities of glycaemic control, BP control, lipid lowering therapy and lifestyle adjustment, more effective treatments for preventing or even halting disease development are needed.

Novel therapeutic strategies which aim to address underlying pathogenesis and potential risk factors of DKD are being developed. Agents interrupting AGEs and its receptor (RAGE), uric acid lowering therapy, and pentoxifylline are under preclinical or clinical research to observe their effects for DKD.[83–85]

Prognosis

People with DKD are at risk of kidney function loss, cardiovascular complications and death, and the prognosis of them is far worse than people with either diabetes or CKD alone. People with DKD have a higher prevalence of atherosclerotic vascular disease, congestive heart failure and death (2- to 3-fold) than those with diabetes and without CKD.[86] People with diabetes and CKD (mainly diabetes-related CKD) have a 13-fold increased relative risk of mortality than those without diabetes.[87]

CVD and ESRD are the major causes of death for DKD. Among people with type 2 diabetes and proteinuria, cardiovascular or non-renal causes account for approximately 90% of death before developing ESRD.[88] For those who develop ESRD, risks of CVD and death are much higher than the general population.[89,90]

References

1. Cheng S, Vijayan A. (2012) The Washington Manual of Nephrology Subspecialty Consult. 3rd ed. Department of Medicine, Washington University School of Medicine.

2. American Diabetes Association. (2015) Microvascular complications and foot care. *Diabetes Care* **38**(Suppl 1): S58–S66.

3. de Boer IH, Rue TC, Hall YN, *et al.* (2011) Temporal Trends in the Prevalence of Diabetic Kidney Disease in the United States. *JAMA* **305**(24): 2532–2539.

4. Loh PT, Toh M, Molina JA, Vathsala A. (2015) Ethnic disparity in prevalence of diabetic kidney disease in an Asian primary healthcare cluster. *Nephrology* **20**(3): 216–223.

5. White S, Chadban S. (2014) KinD Reports (Kidneys in Diabeties): Temporal trends in the epidemiology of diabetic kidney disease and the associated health care burden in Australia. Kidney Health Australia.

6. International Diabetes Federation. (2015) IDF Diabetes Atlas, 7th ed. Brussels, Belgium.

7. Kainz A, Hronsky M, Stel VS, *et al.* (2015) Prediction of prevalence of chronic kidney disease in diabetic patients in countries of the European Union up to 2025. *Nephrol Dial Transplant* **30**: 113–118.

8. Young BA, Katon WJ, Von Korff N, *et al.* (2005) Racial and ethnic differences in microalbuminuria prevalence in a diabetes population: The pathways study. *Clin J Am Soc Nephrol* **16**(1): 219–228.

9. Jia WP, Gao X, Pang C, *et al.* (2009) Prevalence and risk factors of albuminuria and chronic kidney disease in Chinese population with type 2 diabetes and impaired glucose regulation: Shanghai diabetic complications study (SHDCS). *Nephrol Dial Transplant* **24**(12): 3724–3731.

10. Yang CW, Park JT, Kim YS, *et al.* (2011) Prevalence of diabetic nephropathy in primary care type 2 diabetic patients with hypertension: Data from the Korean Epidemiology Study on Hypertension III (KEY III study). *Nephrol Dial Transplant* **26**(10): 3249–3255.

11. Hall V, Thomsen RW, Henriksen O, Lohse N. (2011) Diabetes in Sub Saharan Africa 1999–2011: Epidemiology and public health implications. A systematic review. *BMC Public Health* **11**: 564.

12. da Silva PM, Carvalho D, Nazare J, *et al.* (2015) Prevalence of microalbuminuria in hypertensive patients with or without type 2 diabetes in a Portuguese primary care setting: The RACE (micRoAlbumin sCreening survEy) study. *Revista Portuguesa De Cardiologia* **34**(4): 237–246.

13. National Institutes of Health, National Institute of Diabetes and Digestive and Kidney Diseases. (2014) United States Renal Data System annual data report: Epidemiology of kidney disease in the United States.

14. McDonald S. (2006) The 28th annual report: ANZDATA Australia and New Zealand dialysis and transplant registry. Australia and New Zealand dialysis and transplant registry.
15. Afkarian M, Sachs MC, Kestenbaum B, *et al.* (2013) Kidney disease and increased mortality risk in type 2 diabetes. *Clin J Am Soc Nephrol* **24**(2): 302–308.
16. Global Burden of Disease 2013 Mortality and Causes of Death Collaborators. (2015) Global, regional, and national age-sex specific all-cause and cause-specific mortality for 240 causes of death, 1990–2013: A systematic analysis for the Global Burden of Disease Study 2013. *Lancet* **10**;385(9963): 117–171.
17. White S, Chadban S. (2014) Diabetic kidney disease in Australia: Current burden and future projections. *Nephrology* **19**(8): 450–458.
18. MacIsaac RJ, Ekinci EI, Jerums G. (2014) Markers of and Risk Factors for the Development and Progression of Diabetic Kidney Disease. *Am J Kidney Dis* **63**(2): S39–S62.
19. Mehler PS, Jeffers BW, Biggerstaff SL, Schrier RW. (1998) Smoking as a risk factor for nephropathy in non-insulin-dependent diabetics. *J Gen Intern Med* **13**(12): 842–845.
20. Saiki A, Nagayama D, Ohhira M, *et al.* (2005) Effect of weight loss using formula diet on renal function in obese patients with diabetic nephropathy. *Int J Obes* **29**(9): 1115–1120.
21. Aggarwal J, Kumar M. (2014) Prevalence of Microalbuminuria among Rural North Indian Population with Diabetes Mellitus and its Correlation with Glycosylated Haemoglobin and Smoking. *J Clin Diagn Res* **8**(7): CC11–3.
22. Mann JFE, Gerstein HC, Yi Q-L, *et al.* (2003) Development of Renal Disease in People at High Cardiovascular Risk: Results of the HOPE Randomized Study. *J Am Soc Nephrol* **14**(3): 641–647.
23. Tapp RJ SJ, Zimmet PZ, Balkau B, *et al.* (2004) Albuminuria is evident in the early stages of diabetes onset: Results from the Australian Diabetes, Obesity, and Lifestyle Study (AusDiab). *Am J Kid Dis* **44**(5): 792–798.
24. Cui WP, Du B, Cui YC, *et al.* (2015) Is rs759853 polymorphism in promoter of aldose reductase gene a risk factor for diabetic nephropathy? A meta-analysis. *Eur J Med Res* **20**(1): 14.
25. El-Baz R, Settin A, Ismaeel A, *et al.* (2012) MTHFR C677T, A1298C and ACE I/D polymorphisms as risk factors for diabetic nephropathy among

type 2 diabetic patients. *J Renin Angiotensin Aldosterone Syst* **13**(4): 472–477.

26. Brancati FL WJ, Whelton PK, Seidler AJ, Klag MJ. (1992) The Excess Incidence of Diabetic End-stage Renal Disease Among Blacks. A Population-based Study of Potential Explanatory Factors. *JAMA* **268**(1): 3078–3084.

27. Nelson RG KW, Pettitt DJ, Saad MF, Bennett PH. (1993) Diabetic Kidney Disease in Pima Indians. *Diabetes Care* **16**(1): 335–341.

28. Smith SR SL, Dennis VW. (1991) Racial Differences in the Incidence and Progression of Renal Diseases. *Kidney Int* **40**(5): 815–822.

29. Cao Z, Cooper ME. (2011) Pathogenesis of diabetic nephropathy. *J Diabetes Investing* **2**(4): 243–247.

30. Brownlee M. (2001) Biochemistry and molecular cell biology of diabetic complications. *Nature* **414**(6865): 813–820.

31. Arora MK, Singh UK. (2014) Oxidative stress: Meeting multiple targets in pathogenesis of diabetic nephropathy. *Current Drug Targets* **15**(5): 531–538.

32. Wada J, Makino H. (2013) Inflammation and the pathogenesis of diabetic nephropathy. *Clin Sci* **124**(3): 139–152.

33. Ruggenenti P, Cravedi P, Remuzzi G. (2010) The RAAS in the pathogenesis and treatment of diabetic nephropathy. *Nat Rev Nephrol* **6**(6): 319–330.

34. Adler S. (2004) Diabetic nephropathy: Linking histology, cell biology, and genetics. *Kidney Int* **66**(5): 2095–2106.

35. Fioretto P, Steffes MW, Brown DM, Mauer SM. (1992) An overview of renal pathology in insulin-dependent diabetes mellitus in relationship to altered glomerular hemodynamics. *Am J Kid Dis* **20**(6): 549–558.

36. Kimmelstiel P, Wilson C. (1936) Intercapillary lesions in the glomeruli of the kidney. *Am J Pathol* **12**(1): 83–U30.

37. Tervaert TW, Mooyaart AL, Amann K, *et al.* (2010) Pathologic classification of diabetic nephropathy. *J Am Soc Nephrol* **21**(4): 556–563.

38. Rogers K. (2015) *Diabetic Nephropathy.* Britannica Academic: Encyclopædia Britannica Inc.

39. Levin A, Rocco M. (2007) KDOQI clinical practice guidelines and clinical practice recommendations for diabetes and chronic kidney disease. *Am J Kid Dis* **49**(2): S10–S179.

40. Afkarian M, Zelnick LR, Hall YN, *et al.* (2016) Clinical Manifestations of Kidney Disease Among US Adults With Diabetes, 1988–2014. *JAMA* **316**(6): 602–610.

41. MacIsaac RJ TC, Panagiotopoulos S, Smith TJ, *et al.* (2004) Nonalbuminuric renal insufficiency in Type 2 diabetes. *Diabetes Care* **27**:195–200.

42. Robles NR, Villa J, Gallego RH. (2015) Non-proteinuric Diabetic nephropathy. *J Clin Med* **4**(9): 1761–1773.

43. 中华医学会糖尿病学分会微血管并发症学组. 糖尿病肾病防治专家共识(2014年版). 中华糖尿病杂志, 2014, (11): 792–801.

44. DynaMed Plus. Diabetic nephropathy [Available from: http://www. dynamed.com/topics/dmp~AN~T113702/Diabetic-nephropathy].

45. Lewis G, Maxwell AP. (2014) Risk factor control is key in diabetic nephropathy. *Practitioner* **258**(1768): 13–17.

46. UK Prospective Diabetes Study (UKPDS) Group. (1998) Intensive blood-glucose control with sulphonylureas or insulin compared with conventional treatment and risk of complications in patients with type 2 diabetes (UKPDS 33). *Lancet* **352**(9131): 837–853.

47. de Boer IH, Sun W, Cleary PA, *et al.* (2011) Intensive Diabetes Therapy and Glomerular Filtration Rate in Type 1 Diabetes. *NEJM* **365**(25): 2366–2376.

48. Shamoon H, Duffy H, Fleischer N, *et al.* (1993) The effect of intensive treatment of diabetes on the development and progression of long-term complications in insulin-dependent diabetes-mellitus. *NEJM* **329**(14): 977–986.

49. Tonna S, El-Osta A, Cooper ME, Tikellis C. (2010) Metabolic memory and diabetic nephropathy: Potential role for epigenetic mechanisms. *Nat Rev Nephrol* **6**(6): 332–341.

50. National Kidney Foundation. (2012) KDOQI Clinical Practice Guideline for Diabetes and CKD: 2012 Update. *Am J Kid Dis* **60**(5): 850–886.

51. Advance Collaborative Group, Patel A, MacMahon S, *et al.* (2008) Intensive blood glucose control and vascular outcomes in patients with type 2 diabetes. *NEJM* **358**(24): 2560–2572.

52. Duckworth W, Abraira C, Moritz T, *et al.* (2009) Glucose control and vascular complications in veterans with type 2 diabetes. *NEJM* **360**(2): 129–139.

53. Molitch ME, Adler AI, Flyvbjerg A, *et al.* (2015) Diabetic kidney disease: A clinical update from Kidney Disease: Improving Global Outcomes. *Kidney Int* **87**(1): 20–30.

54. Zanchi A, Lehmann R, Philippe J. (2012) Antidiabetic drugs and kidney disease — recommendations of the Swiss Society for Endocrinology and Diabetology. *Swiss Med Weekly* **142**: w13629.

55. 中国医师协会内分泌代谢科医师分会. 2 型糖尿病合并慢性肾脏病患者口服降糖药用药原则中国专家共识. 中华内分泌代谢杂志, 2016, **32**(6): 455–460.

56. Colhoun HM, Lee ET, Bennett PH, *et al.* (2001) Risk factors for renal failure: The WHO multinational study of vascular disease in diabetes. *Diabetologia* **44**: S46–S53.

57. Ravid M, Brosh D, Ravid-Safran S, *et al.* (1998) Main risk factors for nephropathy in type 2 diabetes mellitus are plasma cholesterol levels, mean blood pressure, and hyperglycemia. *Arch Intern Med* **158**(9): 998–1004.

58. Atkins RC, Briganti EM, Lewis JB, *et al.* (2005) Proteinuria reduction and progression to renal failure in patients with type 2 diabetes mellitus and overt nephropathy. *Am J Kid Dis* **45**(2): 281–287.

59. Brenner BM, Cooper ME, de Zeeuw D, *et al.* (2001) Effects of losartan on renal and cardiovascular outcomes in patients with type 2 diabetes and nephropathy. *NEJM* **345**(12): 861–869.

60. Lewis EJ, Hunsicker LG, Bain RP, Rohde RD. (1993) The effect of angiotensin-converting enzyme-inhibition on diabetic nephropathy. *NEJM* **329**(20): 1456–1462.

61. Lewis EJ, Hunsicker LG, Clarke WR, *et al.* (2001) Renoprotective effect of the angiotensin-receptor antagonist irbesartan in patients with nephropathy due to type 2 diabetes. *NEJM* **345**(12): 851–860.

62. Lv J, Perkovic V, Foote CV, *et al.* (2012) Antihypertensive agents for preventing diabetic kidney disease. *Cochrane Database Syst Rev* **12**: CD004136.

63. Strippoli GF, Bonifati C, Craig M, *et al.* (2006) Angiotensin converting enzyme inhibitors and angiotensin II receptor antagonists for preventing the progression of diabetic kidney disease. *Cochrane Database Syst Rev* **4**: CD006257.

64. Haller H, Ito S, Izzo JL, Jr., *et al.* (2011) Olmesartan for the Delay or Prevention of Microalbuminuria in Type 2 Diabetes. *NEJM* **364**(10): 907–917.

65. Palmer SC, Mavridis D, Navarese E, *et al.* (2015) Comparative efficacy and safety of blood pressure-lowering agents in adults with diabetes and kidney disease: a network meta-analysis. *Lancet* **385**(9982): 2047–2056.

66. Fried LF, Emanuele N, Zhang JH, *et al.* (2013) Combined Angiotensin Inhibition for the Treatment of Diabetic Nephropathy. *NEJM* **369**(20): 1892–1903.

67. Quiroga B, Fernandez Juarez G, Luno J. (2014) Combined Angiotensin Inhibition in Diabetic Nephropathy. *NEJM* **370**(8): 777.

68. Best M, de Wever J, Smulders Y. (2014) Combined Angiotensin Inhibition in Diabetic Nephropathy. *NEJM* **370**(8): 778.

69. Izumi Y, Kawahara K, Nonoguchi H. (2014) Combined Angiotensin Inhibition in Diabetic Nephropathy. *NEJM* **370**(8): 777–778.

70. Nikolaidou B, Lazaridis A, Doumas M. (2014) Combined Angiotensin Inhibition in Diabetic Nephropathy. *NEJM* **370**(8): 778–779.

71. KDIGO Clinical Practice Guideline for the Management of Blood Pressure in Chronic Kidney Disease. (2012) *Kidney Int Suppl* **2**(5): 337–414.

72. Bakris GL, Copley JB, Vicknair N, *et al.* (1996) Calcium channel blockers versus other antihypertensive therapies on progression of NIDDM associated nephropathy. *Kidney Int* **50**(5): 1641–1650.

73. Bakris GL, Toto RD, McCullough PA, *et al.* (2008) Effects of different ACE inhibitor combinations on albuminuria: Results of the GUARD study. *Kidney Int* **73**(11): 1303–1309.

74. Liu LC SE, Gansevoort RT, van der Meer P, Voors AA. (2015) Finerenone: Third-generation Mineralocorticoid Receptor Antagonist for the Treatment of Heart Failure and Diabetic Kidney Disease. *Expert Opin Investig Drugs* **24**(8): 1123–1135.

75. Bakris GL, Agarwal R, Chan JC, *et al.* (2015) Effect of Finerenone on Albuminuria in Patients With Diabetic Nephropathy A Randomized Clinical Trial. *JAMA* **314**(9): 884–894.

76. Jenkins AJ, Lyons TJ, Zheng D, *et al.* (2003) Serum lipoproteins in the diabetes control and complications trial/epidemiology of diabetes intervention and complications cohort: Associations with gender and glycemia. *Diabetes Care* **26**(3): 810–808.

77. Morton J, Zoungas S, Li Q, *et al.* (2012) Low HDL cholesterol and the risk of diabetic nephropathy and retinopathy: Results of the ADVANCE study. *Diabetes Care* **35**(11): 2201–2206.

78. Tolonen N, Forsblom C, Thorn L, *et al.* (2009) Lipid abnormalities predict progression of renal disease in patients with type 1 diabetes. *Diabetologia* **52**(12): 2522–2530.

79. Baigent C, Landray MJ, Reith C, *et al.* (2011) The effects of lowering LDL cholesterol with simvastatin plus ezetimibe in patients with chronic kidney disease (Study of Heart and Renal Protection): A randomised placebo-controlled trial. *Lancet* **377**(9784): 2181–2192.

80. Palmer SC, Navaneethan SD, Craig JC, *et al.* (2014) HMG CoA reductase inhibitors (statins) for people with chronic kidney disease not requiring dialysis. *Cochrane Database Syst Rev* **5**: CD007784.
81. Gaede P, Lund-Andersen H, Parving HH, Pedersen O. (2008) Effect of a multifactorial intervention on mortality in type 2 diabetes. *NEJM* **358**(6): 580–591.
82. Ismail-Beigi F, Craven TE, O'Connor PJ, *et al.* (2012) Combined intensive blood pressure and glycaemic control does not produce an additive benefit on microvascular outcomes in type 2 diabetic patients. *Kidney Int* **81**(6): 586–594.
83. Dwyer JP, Greco BA, Umanath K, *et al.* (2015) Pyridoxamine dihydrochloride in diabetic nephropathy (PIONEER-CSG-17): Lessons learned from a pilot study. *Nephron* **129**(1): 22–28.
84. Hovind P, Rossing P, Johnson R, Parving H. (2011) Serum Uric Acid as a New Player in the Development of Diabetic Nephropathy. *J Renal Nutri* **21**(1): 124–127.
85. McCormick BB, Sydor A, Akbari A, *et al.* (2008) The effect of pentoxifylline on proteinuria in diabetic kidney disease: A meta-analysis. *Am J Kidney Dis* **52**(3): 454–463.
86. Foley RN, Murray AM, Li S, *et al.* (2005) Chronic kidney disease and the risk for cardiovascular disease, renal replacement, and death in the United States Medicare population, 1998 to 1999. *J Am Soc Nephrol* **16**(2): 489–495.
87. Bragg F, Holmes MV, Iona A, *et al.* (2017) Association Between Diabetes and Cause-Specific Mortality in Rural and Urban Areas of China. *JAMA* **317**(3): 280–289.
88. Taal MW CG, Marsden PA, Skorecki K, *et al.* (2011) Brenner and *Rector's The Kidney E-Book*: Elsevier Health Sciences.
89. Longenecker JC, Coresh J, Powe NR, *et al.* (2002) Traditional cardiovascular disease risk factors in dialysis patients compared with the general population: the CHOICE Study. *JASN* **13**(7): 1918–1927.
90. Groop PH, Thomas MC, Moran JL, *et al.* (2009) The presence and severity of chronic kidney disease predicts all-cause mortality in type 1 diabetes. *Diabetes* **58**(7):1651–1658.

2

Diabetic Kidney Disease in Chinese Medicine

OVERVIEW

Symptom descriptions corresponding to diabetic kidney disease (DKD) can be found in ancient Chinese medicine (CM) literature. Based on CM theory, DKD is a deficient condition with excess pathogen, and the deficiency may involve *yin, yang, qi* and/or Blood. DKD mainly affects the Kidney, as well as the Lung, Liver and Spleen. This chapter introduces CM treatments including Chinese herbal medicine, acupuncture and other CM therapies such as exercise and diet therapy for DKD recommended by CM guidelines or specialist monographs.

Introduction

Diabetic kidney disease (DKD) is a modern disease definition based on pathological changes in the kidneys leading to albuminuria and progressive loss of kidney function. DKD is not mentioned in the ancient Chinese medical literature. However, a large number of citations mention symptoms and signs similar to DKD, including the terms *Xiao ke* 消渴 (diabetes), *Xiao dan* 消瘅 (diabetes), *San xiao* 三消 (diabetes), *Shui zhong* 水肿 (oedema), *Niao zhuo* 尿浊 (turbid urine), *Guan ge* 关格 (oliguria and vomiting), *Xu lao* 虚劳 (consumption), *Shen xiao* 肾消 (kidney injury), *Xiao shen* 消肾 (kidney injury) and *Xia xiao* 下消 (kidney injury).

Scholars have attempted to trace the origins of DKD in ancient Chinese language and literature. They suggest that although highly similar clinical descriptions were seen in the ancient citations such as

Shui zhong 水肿, *Niao zhuo* 尿浊, *Guan ge* 关格, *Xu lao* 虚劳 and *Shen lao* 肾劳, these terms were not specific enough to represent DKD if not accompanied by a description of diabetic history. Two ancient disease names, *San xiao* 三消 and *Xiao dan* 消瘅, represented the pathogenic process of diabetic kidney injury, therefore the concept of DKD is primarily referred to as these two ancient diseases.[1] As for *Xiao shen* 消肾, *Shen xiao* 肾消 and *Xia xiao* 下消, their typical symptoms included muscle dystrophy in the lower half of the body, bone and joint pain, thirst with or without polydipsia, frequent urine with turbid and sweet properties. The clinical manifestations of these three ancient diseases are relatively consistent with DKD as it is known today.[2]

A single ancient disease name is not wholly representative of DKD because the meanings from ancient literature vary based on specific symptoms. Therefore, modern Chinese medicine (CM) disease nomenclature refers to DKD (also diabetic nephropathy) as *"Xiao ke bing shen bing* 消渴病肾病*"* which profiles the various symptoms of DKD.[3]

Aetiology and Pathogenesis

Constitutional insufficiency of the five *zang* organs, especially Kidney deficiency, is the internal cause of DKD, as *Miraculous Pivot* 灵枢 says "People with five *zang* organs deficiency are vulnerable to *Xiao dan* 消瘅." Dietary irregularities and alcohol addiction may also trigger DKD, as *Peaceful Holy Benevolent Prescriptions* 太平圣惠方 accounts "*San xiao* 三消 is rooted from constitutional Kidney deficiency or daily unhealthy greasy food intake." In addition, emotional disorders, internal damage caused by overexertion and fatigue, erroneous treatment, or overconsumption of medicinal agents with warm and dry properties may also cause DKD.[4]

Generally, DKD is characterised as root deficiency with accompanied excess. Root deficiency mainly refers to Kidney deficiency and debilitation of *yin, yang, qi* and Blood, while excess involves abnormalities including stasis obstructing the Kidney collateral, internal water-dampness and turbid toxin due to deficient healthy *qi*. In addition to the Kidney, DKD also affects the Lung, Liver and Spleen.[5–7]

The pathogenesis of DKD generally follows the following pattern: Kidney deficiency internally engenders dryness-heat pathogen, which depletes fluid and humour. Subsequent detriment to *yin* affects *yang*, developing into dual damage of *yin* and *yang*. As for symptoms, these vary in different stages. In the early stage, patients may feel thirsty even with excess fluid intake, fatigue, lack of strength, dry eyes with blurred vision, or numbness of the limbs. These symptoms appear as dryness-heat depleting *qi* and *yin*, and if they persist, they further deprive *zang* organs and meridians of nourishment. As the disease progresses, the five *zang* organs continue to be damaged affecting the Kidney. Damage to Kidney *yang* causes essence depletion and impedes the Kidney downward draining function, which symptomatically produces turbid urine. Abnormal Kidney *qi* transforms into internal water-dampness retention causing oedema. In the advanced stage, debilitation of *qi*, Blood, *yin* and *yang*, and congestion of dampness turbidity and static Blood, the symptoms of oliguria, pitting oedema, nausea or vomiting (*Guan ge* 关格 and *Long bi* 癃闭) are observed.[5–7]

Syndrome Differentiation and Treatments

The fundamental therapeutic principles of DKD are to treat the deficiency as well as the excess. In the early stage, patterns of Liver-Kidney *yin* deficiency or dual deficiency of *qi* and *yin*, usually combined with internal heat, Blood stasis, or phlegm turbidity, are common. As DKD progresses, Spleen-Kidney *yang* deficiency, and dual deficiency of *qi* and Blood coexist with internally retained dampness turbidity and stasis toxin. Consequently, syndromes at different stages will have varying treatments. For instance, early treatment should focus on nourishing *yin*, tonifying *qi*, clearing heat, and activating Blood. In the moderate or advanced stages, treatment should focus on securing Kidney *yang*, with methods including draining water, dispelling stasis, and expelling toxin.

Chinese medicine (CM) treatments for DKD include Chinese herbal medicine (CHM), multi-herb or single-herb formulae based on syndrome differentiation, acupuncture, other CM treatments and integrative treatments of CM and conventional medicine. In the early stages of DKD, CHM may be used alone but, as DKD progresses, the effects of CHM alone may be less potent especially when the patterns include turbidity toxin obstruction and dual deficiency of *yin* and *yang*. Optimal treatment in advanced disease therefore includes integrative use of CM and conventional medicine.

Multiple clinical practice guidelines on nephrologic diagnosis and treatment in CM were used as references in the following section. They include:

- Chinese medicine diagnosis and treatments standards for diabetic kidney disease (糖尿病肾脏疾病中医诊疗标准) published by the China Association of Chinese Medicine Diabetes Branch.[7]
- Diagnosis, syndrome classification and effect evaluation standards for diabetic kidney disease (糖尿病肾病诊断、辨证分型及疗效评定标准) published by the China Association of Chinese Medicine Nephropathy Branch.[8]
- Chinese medicine clinical diagnosis and treatment strategy (糖尿病中医防治指南—糖尿病肾病) published by the China Association of Chinese Medicine.[9]
- Evidence-based guidelines of clinical practice in Chinese medicine: Internal medicine (中医循证临床实践指南—中医内科) published by the China Academy of Chinese Medical Sciences.[11]
- Integrative Chinese and Western Medicine (中西医结合内科学) written by Guangxian Cai 蔡光先 and Yuyong Zhao 赵玉庸.[12]
- Internal Chinese medicine (中医内科学) written by Keji Chen 陈可冀.[13]

It should be noted that the use of some herbs, such as *fu zi* 附子, may be restricted in some countries. In addition, some herbs, such as *shui zhi* 水蛭, are restricted under the provisions of the Convention on International Trade in Endangered Species of Wild Fauna and Flora (CITES). Readers are advised to comply with relevant regulations.

Chinese Herbal Medicine Treatment Based on Syndrome

Deficiency Syndromes

Dual deficiency of *qi* and *yin*

Clinical manifestations: turbid urine, drowsiness, fatigue, shortness of breath, lazy speech, dry mouth and throat, dizziness, dreaming, frequent urination with copious urine, heat in the palms and soles, palpitations and agitation, (pale) red thin shrunken tongue with scanty dry coat, and sunken weak pulse.[13]

Treatment principle: Tonifying *qi* and *yin.*

Formula: *Shen qi di huang tang*[14] 参芪地黄汤

Herbs: *dang shen* 党参, *huang qi* 黄芪, *fu ling* 茯苓, *shu di huang* 熟地黄, *shan yao* 山药, *shan zhu yu* 山茱萸, *mu dan pi* 牡丹皮, *ze xie* 泽泻

Main actions of herbs: *Dang shen* and *huang qi* tonify *qi* and fortify the Spleen. Accompanied with *Liu wei di huang wan* 六味地黄丸 (*fu ling, shu di huang, shan yao, shan zhu yu, mu dan pi, ze xie*) to enrich the Kidney and nourish the Liver.

Liver-Kidney *yin* deficiency

Clinical manifestations: turbid urine, dizziness, tinnitus, vexing heat in the chest, palms and soles, aching back and knees, dry eyes, short voiding of scanty urine, red tongue with scant coat, and fine rapid pulse.[13]

Treatment principle: Enrich the Kidney and nourish the Liver.

Formula: *Qi ju di huang wan*[15] 杞菊地黄丸

Herbs: *gou qi zi* 枸杞子, *ju hua* 菊花, *shu di huang* 熟地黄, *shan zhu yu* 山茱萸, *shan yao* 山药, *fu ling* 茯苓, *ze xie* 泽泻, *mu dan pi* 牡丹皮

Main actions of herbs: *Gou qi zi* emolliates the Liver, tonifies the Kidney and replenishes essence. *Ju hua* dispels Liver heat. All herbs act together and nourish *yin,* emolliate the Liver, tonify the Kidney and replenish essence.

Dual deficiency of *qi* and Blood

Clinical manifestations: turbid urine, fatigue, shortness of breath, lazy speech, pale or sallow complexion, blurred vision accompanied by vertigo, pale lips and nails, palpitations, insomnia, aching back and knees, pale tongue, and weak pulse.[13]

Treatment principle: Tonify *qi* and Blood.

Formula: *Dang gui bu xue tang*[16] 当归补血汤 combined with *Ji sheng shen qi wan*[17] 济生肾气丸

Herbs: *huang qi* 黄芪, *dang gui* 当归, *fu zi* 附子, *rou gui* 肉桂, *shu di huang* 熟地黄, *shan yao* 山药, *shan zhu yu* 山茱萸, *fu ling* 茯苓, *mu dan pi* 牡丹皮, *ze xie* 泽泻, *che qian zi* 车前子, *niu xi* 牛膝

Main actions of herbs: *Dang gui bu xue tang: huang qi* tonifies healthy *qi*, and *dang gui* tonifies Blood and harmonises nutrients to engender *qi* and Blood. Together with *Ji sheng shen qi wan*, it warms the Kidney and induces diuresis to alleviate oedema.

Spleen-Kidney *yang* deficiency

Clinical manifestations: turbid urine, fatigue, lack of mental vigour, fear of cold, cold aching back and knees, puffy swollen limbs (particularly lower limbs), pale complexion, frequent and excessive volume of urination, increased nocturnal urine, diarrhoea at dawn, pale enlarged tongue with teeth marks, and sunken slow forceless pulse.[13]

Treatment principle: Warm the Kidney and fortify the Spleen.

Formula: *Fu zi li zhong wan*[18] 附子理中丸 combined with *Zhen wu tang*[19] 合真武汤

Herbs: *fu zi* 附子, *sheng jiang* 生姜, *dang shen* 党参, *bai zhu* 白术, *fu ling* 茯苓, *bai shao* 白芍, *gan cao* 甘草

Main actions of herbs: *Fu zi* warms the Kidney and Spleen. *Fu ling* and *bai zhu* tonify *qi* and fortify the Spleen and induce diuresis to drain dampness. *Sheng jiang* warms *yang* and dissipates water *qi*, and *bai shao* constrains *yin* and prevents dryness.

Dual deficiency of *yin* and *yang*

Clinical manifestations: soot-black complexion, fear of cold and cold limbs, frequent urination, turbid urine, aching back and knees, impotence or menstrual irregularities, dry mouth with desire to drink, oedema, dry or thin stool, pale dark or red tongue with white coat, and sunken fine forceless pulse.[13]

Treatment principle: Tonify both *yin* and *yang*.

Formula: *Jin gui shen qi wan*[20] 金匮肾气丸

Herbs: *gui zhi* 桂枝, *fu zi* 附子, *shan yao* 山药, *shan zhu yu* 山茱萸, *shu di huang* 熟地黄, *fu ling* 茯苓, *ze xie* 泽泻, *mu dan pi* 牡丹皮.

Main actions of herbs: *Shu di huang* nourishes Kidney *yin*. *Shan zhu yu* tonifies the Kidney and astringes essence. *Shan yao* fortifies the Spleen and the Kidney, and secures essence. *Gui zhi* and *fu zi* warms the Kidney and tonifies *yang*. *Fu ling* fortifies the Spleen, tonifies the Kidney, drains dampness and discharges turbidity. *Ze xie* and *mu dan pi* suppress the hyperactive ministerial fire.

Excess Syndromes

Blood stasis

Clinical manifestations: numbness and pain in the limbs, dark purple lips, sublingual varices, dark purple tongue with or without stasis speckles and stasis macules, and sunken rough string-like pulse.

Herbs: Add Blood-activating and stasis-resolving herbs including *dang gui* 当归, *tao ren* 桃仁, *hong hua* 红花, *chuan xiong* 川芎, or *dan shen* 丹参 to the formulae for deficiency syndromes.

Dampness turbidity

Clinical manifestations: distention and fullness feeling in the stomach and abdomen, indigestion, loss of appetite, nausea, thin sloppy stool, heavy cumbersome limbs, and thin slimy tongue coat plus symptoms of deficiency syndromes.

Herbs: Add dampness-turbidity-resolving herbs including *ban xia* 半夏, *fu ling* 茯苓 or *chen pi* 陈皮 to the formulae for deficiency syndromes.

Manufactured CHM Treatments

Bailing capsules[11,20]

Composition: powdered *dong chong xia cao* 冬虫夏草 (drying mycelium power made from *Cs-C-Q8Hirsutella sinensis Liu, Guo, Yu-et Zeng 1989*, submerged fermentation).

Indications: This formulation is designed to tonify the Lung and Kidney. It is indicated for patients with DKD in the early and moderate stage with dual deficiency of Lung and Kidney syndrome.

Dosage and administration: 3g (6 capsules) to be administered orally three times per day.

Jin shui bao capsules[7,21]

Composition: fermented *dong chong xia cao* 冬虫夏草 *Cordyceps sinensis* (Berk.) Sacc. (*Cs-4*) powder.

Indications: This formulation is designed to tonify the Spleen-Kidney, and essence-*qi*. It is indicated for patients with DKD with Lung-Kidney *qi* deficiency syndrome.

Dosage and administration: 0.99g (3 capsules) to be administered orally three times per day.

Huang kui capsules[7]

Composition: *huang shu kui hua* 黄蜀葵花 *Abelmoschus Manihot* (L.) Medic. flower.

Indications: This formulation is designed for clearing heat, draining dampness, resolving toxin, and dispersing oedema. It is indicated for patients with DKD with dampness-heat syndrome and pitting oedema.

Contraindication: Pregnancy.

Dosage and administration: 2.5g (5 capsules) to be administered orally three times per day.

Qi zhi jiang tang capsule[7,21]

Composition: *huang qi* 黄芪, *di huang* 地黄, *huang jing* 黄精, *shui zhi* 水蛭.

Indications: This formulation is designed to tonify *qi*, nourish *yin*, activate Blood and resolve stasis. It is indicated for patients with DKD with dual deficiency of *qi* and *yin* syndrome with concurrent Blood stasis.

Contraindications: It is contraindicated in pregnancy, and should not be used in patients with coagulation disorders or bleeding tendency.

Dosage and administration: 2g (4 capsules) to be administered orally three times per day.

Herbal Retention Enema

Herbal retention enema is indicated for moderate or advanced DKD patients with Spleen-Kidney deficiency prior to turbidity toxin retention which invades the Spleen and Stomach.[7,11] Such patients may manifest with symptoms of nausea, turbidity in the mouth, constipation, and yellowish-brown urine. Herbs including *sheng da huang* 生大黄, *pu gong ying* 蒲公英, *sheng mu li* 生牡蛎, *dan shen* 丹参 are optimal for treatment. *Huang qi* 黄芪 or *fu zi* 附子 could be additionally used for patients with combined *yang* deficiency syndrome. Prescribed formula should be decocted with water to 100–200ml extract, and then cooled down to 36°C. It is then used for 30-minute as a retention enema once or twice per day depending on the patients' frequency of defecation. Note that this treatment is not common outside of China.

Acupuncture Therapies and Other Chinese Medicine Therapies

Selection of acupuncture points should be according to the patients' CM syndrome and DKD stage. Common acupuncture points and corresponding needle manipulation are as follows[7]:

- Dual deficiency of *qi* and *yin*
  Acupoints: supplementation manipulation of BL23 *Shenshu* 肾俞, BL20 *Pishu* 脾俞, ST36 *Zusanli* 足三里, SP6 *Sanyinjiao* 三阴交, BL52 *Zhishi* 志室, KI3 *Taixi* 太溪, KI7 *Fuliu* 复溜, CV2 *Qugu* 曲骨; reducing manipulation of LR2 *Xingjian* 行间.

- Liver-Kidney *yin* deficiency
  Acupoints: supplementation manipulation of BL18 *Ganshu* 肝俞, BL23 *Shenshu* 肾俞, LR14 *Qimen* 期门, BL40 *Weizhong* 委中.

- Spleen-Kidney *yang* deficiency
  Acupoints: supplementation manipulation of BL20 *Pishu* 脾俞, BL23 *Shenshu* 肾俞, GV4 *Mingmen* 命门, SP6 *Sanyinjiao* 三阴交, KI3 *Taixi* 太溪, CV3 *Zhongji* 中极, CV4 *Guanyuan* 关元.

- Dual deficiency of *yin* and *yang*
  Acupoints: supplementation manipulation of BL20 *Pishu* 脾俞, BL23 *Shenshu* 肾俞, GV4 *Mingmen* 命门, SP6 *Sanyinjiao* 三阴交, CV6 *Qihai* 气海, CV4 *Guanyuan* 关元.

Needle manipulation should be cautiously practiced on DKD patients with serious oedema to prevent potential local exudation and infection.

Ear Acupressure is also used for DKD In China, *wang bu liu xing* 王不留行籽, *Vaccaria segetalis* seeds are attached to the ear points.[22] Other instruments such as stainless steel beads or magnets may be used in China but are more commonly used outside China.[23] The points can be pressed three to five times per ear, per day, three to five minutes each time.[22] Common ear points for DKD include: Gallbladder CO11 胰胆, Kidney CO10 肾, *San Jiao* CO17 三焦, and Endocrine CO18 内分泌.

Other Management Strategies

Lifestyle modification: Lifestyle modifications are suggested, including smoking cessation, weight management and physical exercise. Moderate intensity exercise (such as *Tai chi* 太极, *Ba duan jin* 八段锦

and walking) with proper rest is suitable for patients in the early stages of DKD. However, in advanced stages of DKD, especially in the stage of kidney failure, overexertion is not recommended. For these patients, *qi* cultivation, *qi*-Blood harmonisation, and dredging the meridian is beneficial. This can be achieved through *Qi gong* 气功, deep breathing, and meditation, etc.[5,7,9]

Diet therapy: CM diet therapy may be beneficial. This depends on an individuals' constitution, disease progression and their CM syndrome differentiation.[7] CM diet recipes are presented in Table 2.1 for reference.

Table 2.1. Chinese Medicine Diet Recipes for Diabetic Kidney Disease

Syndrome Differentiation	Chinese Medicine Diet Name	Recipe
Kidney *yang* deficiency	NA	*rou gui* 肉桂
Kidney *yin* deficiency	NA	*gou qi* 枸杞, *sang shen zi* 桑葚子, *yin er* 银耳
Spleen deficiency	NA	*bian dou* 扁豆, *yi yi ren* 薏苡仁, *shan yao* 山药, *lian zi* 莲子
Spleen deficiency accompany oedema	*Yi yi ren zhou* 薏苡仁粥	congee with *yi yi ren* 薏苡仁 and *jing mi* 粳米
	Huang qi dong gua tang 黄芪冬瓜汤	soup with *huang qi* 黄芪 and *dong gua* 冬瓜
	Qian jin li yu tang 千金鲤鱼汤	soup with 1 carp (fish), *sha ren* 砂仁 (5g), ginger and scallion, no salt
Dual deficiency of the Spleen-Kidney	*Huang qi shan yao zhou* 黄芪山药粥	congee with *huang qi* 黄芪 and *shan yao* 山药

Table reference[4]

Table 2.2.   Summary of Chinese Medicine Treatments for Diabetic Kidney Disease

Syndrome Differentiation	Treatment Principle	Chinese Herbal Medicine (Formula)	Acupuncture	Other Therapy
Dual deficiency of *qi* and *yin*	Tonify *qi* and *yin*	*Shen qi di huang tang* 参芪地黄汤	BL23 *Shenshu* 肾俞, BL20 *Pishu* 脾俞, ST36 *Zusanli* 足三里, SP6 *Sanyinjiao* 三阴交, BL52 *Zhishi* 志室, KI3 *Taixi* 太溪, KI7 *Fuliu* 复溜, CV2 *Qugu* 曲骨, LR2 *Xingjian* 行间	Herbal retention enema for moderate or advanced DKD patients; Lifestyle modification; diet therapy
Liver-Kidney *yin* deficiency	Enrich the Kidney and nourish the Liver	*Qi Ju Di huang Pill* 杞菊地黄丸	BL18 *Ganshu* 肝俞, BL23 *Shenshu* 肾俞, LR14 *Qimen* 期门, BL40 *Weizhong* 委中	
Spleen-Kidney *yang* deficiency	Warm the Kidney and fortify the Spleen	*Fu zi li zhong wan* combined with *Zhen wu tang* 附子理中丸合真武汤	BL20 *Pishu* 脾俞, BL23 *Shenshu* 肾俞, GV4 *Mingmen* 命门, SP6 *Sanyinjiao* 三阴交, KI3 *Taixi* 太溪, CV3 *Zhongji* 中极, CV4 *Guanyuan* 关元	
Dual deficiency of *yin* and *yang*	Tonify *yin* and *yang*	*Jin gui shen qi wan* 金匮肾气丸	BL20 *Pishu* 脾俞, BL23 *Shenshu* 肾俞, GV4 *Mingmen* 命门, SP6 *Sanyinjiao* 三阴交, CV6 *Qihai* 气海, CV4 *Guanyuan* 关元	
Dual deficiency of *qi* and Blood	Tonify *qi* and Blood	*Dang gui bu xue tang* combined with *Ji sheng shen qi wan* 当归补血汤合济生肾气丸	Specific points not recommended. Treatment selected based on point functions.	

References

1. 王庆华. 糖尿病肾病中医相关文献考辨与方药证治规律研究. 广州中医药大学. 2008.
2. 张蕾，刘旭生. 糖尿病肾病中医病名源流探索性研究. 辽宁中医杂志. 2012. (1): 52–54.
3. 吕仁和，赵进喜，王越. 糖尿病肾病临床研究述评. 北京中医药大学学报. 1994. **19**(2): 2–6.
4. 郑健. 中西医结合肾病学. 北京. 科学出版社. 2011.
5. 中华中医药学会. 糖尿病肾病中医防治指南. 中国中医药现代远程教育. 2011; **9**(4): 151–153.
6. 沈庆发. 中医肾病学. 上海. 上海中医药大学. 2007.
7. 中华中医药学会糖尿病分会. 糖尿病肾脏疾病中医诊疗标准. 世界中西医结合杂志. 2011. **6**(6): 548–552.
8. 中华中医药学会肾病分会. 糖尿病肾病诊断、辨证分型及疗效评定标准 (试行方案). 上海中医药杂志. 2007. **41**(7): 7–8.
9. 中华中医药学会. 糖尿病中医防治指南. 北京, 中国中医药出版社, 2007.
10. 中国中医科学院. 中医循证临床实践指南 — 中医内科. 北京. 中国中医药出版社. 2011. 95–118.
11. 蔡光先, 赵玉庸. 中西医结合内科学. 北京: 中国中医药出版社. 2005.
12. 陈可冀. 高级医师案头丛书：中医内科学. 北京. 中国协和医科大学出版社. 2002.
13. World Health Organization. WHO International Standard Terminologies on Traditional Medicine in the Western Pacific Region. World Health Organization, Western Pacific Region, Geneva, 2007.
14. 清·沈金鳌. 沈氏尊生书.
15. 清·董西园. 医级.
16. 金·李杲撰. 兰室秘藏.
17. 宋·严用和. 济生方.
18. 宋·陈师文，太平惠民和剂局. 太平惠民和剂局方.
19. 东汉·张仲景. 伤寒论.
20. 东汉·张仲景. 金匮要略.
21. 国家药典委员会. 中华人民共和国药典. 北京. 中国医药科技出版社. 2015.
22. Chen P, Michael H. (2004) *Modern Chinese Ear Acupressure*. Paradigm Publications. Taos, New Mexico.
23. Wang Y. (2009) *Micro-acupuncture in Practice*. Churchill Livingstone, Missouri, USA.

3

Classical Chinese Medicine Literature

OVERVIEW

Classical literature forms the foundation of Chinese medicine knowledge and continues to guide clinical practice. Although the classical literature does not specifically describe diabetic kidney disease (DKD), and laboratory testing of kidney function was not available, the literature does describe groups of symptoms that are characteristic of DKD as it is understood today. This chapter includes findings from a search of the *Zhong Hua Yi Dian* 中华医典 from AD 206 to 1949. Over 1,000 classical books were analysed. Chinese herbal medicine formulae and herbs were commonly used for the treatment of DKD in ancient times.

Introduction

Diabetes and its complications, including diabetic kidney disease (DKD), are described in classical Chinese medicine (CM) literature. Written in the Han dynasty (AD 202–220), the book, *Synopsis of Prescriptions of the Golden Chamber* 金匮要略 recorded cases of patients with renal impairment including polyuria after a long history of diabetes. In the book *Treatise on the Pathogenesis and Manifestations of All Diseases* 诸病源候论 published in the Sui dynasty (AD 581–618), patients with diabetes and frequent urination were grouped as *Nei xiao* 内消 syndrome. Meanwhile, *Shen xiao* disease 肾消 was first recorded in the book *Gu Jin Lu Yan* 古今录验 which described frequent urination with lower limb oedema. Up until the Song dynasty (AD 960–1279), *Xiao shen* 消肾 was used to describe diabetes and renal complications and its aetiology and disease mechanism, was comprehensively documented in the official medical prescription monograph *Peaceful Holy Benevolent Prescriptions* 太平圣惠方. *Xiao shen* 消肾 was regarded as a sub-type of diabetes with renal involvement, belonging to the *Shan xiao* 三消 disease together with *Xiao ke* 消渴 and *Xiao zhong* 消中. After the Jin and Yuan dynasties (after 1368), *Shen xiao* 肾消 and *Xiao shen* 消肾 diseases were both attributed to *Xia xiao* 下消.

In the field of CM, ancient clinical experience for treating DKD was passed down from generation to generation though records in medical books. Therefore, it is of great value to systematically assess the classical literature. In order to obtain a sample of the classical and pre-modern medical literature, we conducted electronic searches of the *Zhong Hua Yi Dian* (ZHYD) 中华医典 *'Encyclopaedia of Traditional Chinese Medicine'*, a CD of more than 1,000 medical books.[1] This collection is the largest currently available and is representative of other large collections of the classical and pre-modern Chinese medical literature.[2–3]

Search Terms

CM disease nomenclatures include a number of traditional disease names of potential relevance to DKD.[4] *Niao zhuo* 尿浊 can refer to 'turbid urine' or 'proteinuria'; and *shui zhong* 水肿 or *shui qi bing* 水气病 refers to 'oedema'; *guan ge* 关格 refers to concurrence of 'anuria' and 'vomit'; *shen lao* 肾劳 refers to symptoms of renal insufficiency. Although these terms and their synonyms refer to disorders involving kidney damage, they are not specific for DKD and can include renal disorders of various aetiologies. The modern CM term *xiao ke bing shen bing* 消渴病肾病 is more specific for DKD and refers to 'kidney damage occurring in diabetes'; however, this term does not appear in the classical literature.[5]

In order to select terms for searching the ZHYD, the classical terms for diabetes and its complications were studied. Textbooks, dictionaries and medical nomenclatures were consulted and a nation-wide questionnaire survey on the historical use of terms for DKD was performed.[4] Classical terms highly rated by experts and based on their consensus were further verified by cross checking their corresponding modern disease definition in textbooks and monographs. Only classical terms with corresponding modern disease definitions which refer to kidney damage occurring in diabetes were included. As a result, the terms identified as most relevant to DKD were *xiao shen* 消肾, *shen xiao* 肾消, *xia xiao* 下消 and these terms were used to search the ZHYD.

Search Procedure and Data Coding

Each search term was entered into the ZHYD search fields and the search results were downloaded to spread sheets. A 'citation' was defined as a distinct passage of text referring to one or more of the search terms. Codes were allocated for types of citations, books and

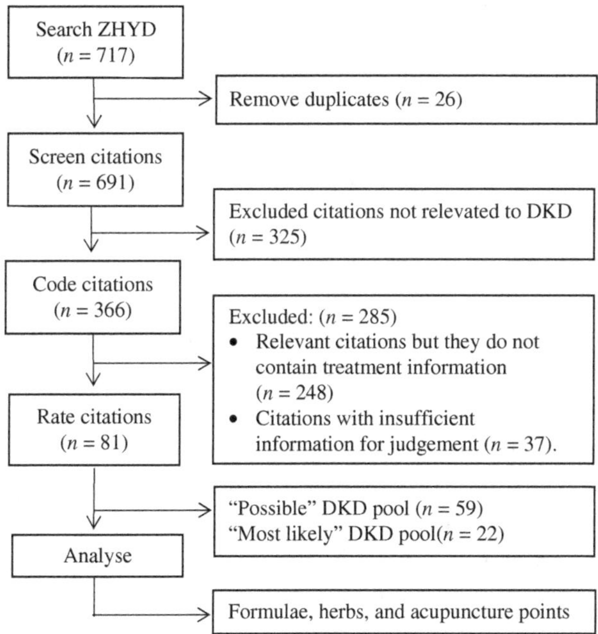

Fig. 3.1. Classical Literature Citations.

Abbreviations: DKD, diabetic kidney disease; ZHYD, *Zhong Hua Yi Dian* "Encyclopedia of Traditional Chinese Medicine".

the dynasties in which they were written according to the procedures described in May *et al.* 2013.[3] Books written after 1949 were excluded.

Data Analysis Procedure

The number of citations identified by each search term was calculated by summing the results of the searches. After removing duplicates, exclusion criteria were then applied to remove citations which were considered not related to DKD (i.e. not relevant) (Fig. 3.1).

Inclusion and Exclusion Criteria

The following exclusion criteria were applied to identify citations that were unlikely to refer to DKD: conditions without symptoms of kidney damage disorders; without symptoms or history or comorbidity of diabetes. Conditions that may have been associated with other kidney diseases, including symptoms such as haematuria, fatigue, nausea, or caused by other aetiologies, such as prostatitis, were identified and excluded from the data set. Citations which contained no information or insufficient information to judge the likelihood of being DKD were also excluded.

All relevant citations were reviewed to identify the best descriptions of DKD and its aetiology or pathogenesis. Experts in DKD and classical literature coded the citations to indicate if they described one or more of the common DKD characteristics including history of diabetes, increased thirst, profuse drinking, increased hunger, weight loss, profuse urine, sweet urine, frequent urination, turbid urine (protein urine), or oedema of the lower limbs. An additional coding process was performed to identify citations considered 'possibly' or 'most likely' DKD (Table 3.1). A judgment of possible DKD was made when citations mentioned a history of diabetes and symptoms of kidney disease or symptoms of diabetes and symptoms of kidney disease. A judgment of most likely DKD was made when citations mentioned a history of diabetes, symptoms of diabetes and symptoms of kidney disease.

Table 3.1. Judgement Criteria for the Likelihood of being Diabetic Kidney Disease

Categories	Criteria
Not Diabetic Kidney Disease	Does not include any symptoms of kidney disease
Conditional DKD	Only includes symptoms of kidney disease
Possible DKD	Includes diabetes history and symptoms of kidney disease or symptoms of diabetes and kidney disease
Most likely DKD	Includes diabetes history and symptoms of kidney disease and symptoms of diabetes

Relevant citations which did not include treatment were excluded from further analysis. Citations which were pharmacopeia-type entries were reviewed for eligibility. Pharmacopeia entries which mentioned the name of the condition but did not include a detailed description of the condition or information about treatment were excluded from further analysis. Pharmacopeia entries which included a description of the condition, with or without reference to other herbs, were included. Single acupuncture points were reviewed in a similar manner. Data are presented as frequencies of identified formulae, herbs and acupuncture points for 'possible' and 'most likely' DKD. When a citation referred to multiple treatments, each treatment was considered as a separate citation for calculation of formulae, herbs, or acupuncture points.

Search Results

A total of 717 classical literature citations contained at least one of the three pre-specified search terms (Table 3.2). The term *xia xiao* 下消 located almost half of the citations (46.9%). The other two search terms, *shen xiao* 肾消 and *xiao shen* 消肾, describing diabetes manifesting as polydipsia, polyuria, frequent urination and turbid urine, contributed similar propotions of citations (26.6% and 26.5%, respectively). The proportions of search term frequency in the possible DKD pool and most likely DKD pool were similar compared to the total pool.

Table 3.2.   Citation Frequency by Search Term

Pinyin	Chinese Characters	Hit Frequency (n, %)		
		Total Pool	Possible Pool	Most Likely Pool
Xia xiao	下消	336(46.9)	11(18.6)	8(36.4)
Shen xiao	肾消	191(26.6)	17(28.8)	8(36.4)
Xiao shen	消肾	190(26.5)	31(52.5)	6(27.3)

After duplicate removal, the remaining citations were coded based on diabetes and kidney disease symptoms, in order to identify the citations consistent with DKD manifestation as it is understood in modern literature. As a result, a total of 366 citations related to DKD including 248 citations describing the disease definition, disease mechanisms and treatment principles. One hundred and sixty (160) citations reported treatments of DKD and these citations were further judged for their likelihood of being DKD. In total, 59 citations were judged as possible DKD and included in the data analysis. Citations were located in 26 different classical books written from AD 652 to 1839. Representative citations related to DKD are listed below.

Citations Related to Diabetic Kidney Disease

In the book *Su Wen Bing Ji Qi Yi Bao Ming Ji* 素问病机气宜保命集 (AD 1186) written by *Liu Wan Su* 刘完素, symptoms, disease progression process, mechanism and treatment principle of *Shen xiao* 肾消 were recorded. It stated that *Shen xiao* 肾消 was one of the complications of diabetes (*Xiao ke* 消渴) and the disease is located in the Kidney. The symptom onset of *Shen xiao* 肾消 includes turbid and frequent urine, as the condition worsens, the facial complexion gradually becomes dark with continuous weight loss. The treatment principle includes nourishing Blood in order to restore the separation of the clear and turbid fluid in the body. "论曰：消渴之疾，三焦受病也。有上消中消肾消…肾消者。病在下焦。初发为膏淋。下如膏油之状。至病成而面色鬡黑。形瘦而耳焦。小便浊而有脂。治法宜养血。以肃清。分其清浊而自愈也。"

In *Bian Que Xin Shu* 扁鹊心书 published on AD 1146, it is stated that *Xiao xia* 下消 was named *Fei xiao* 肺消 in *Plain Questions* 素问 and was defined as thirst, frequent urination with turbid urine. The citation mentioned that at the time, it had recently been defined as *Shen xiao* 肾消, which had been considered as a severe disease stage. As the disease progressed, patients presented with cachexia, weak pulse and sweet urine and they were considered to be in a critical condition. The overall treatment principle was to engender the fluid and humour. "消渴虽有上中下之分，总由于损耗津液所致，盖肾为津液之原，脾为津液之本，本原亏而消渴之证从此致矣…下消者，《素问》谓之肺消，渴而便数有膏。饮一溲二；后人又谓之肾消，肾消之证则已重矣。若脉微而涩或细小，身体瘦瘁，溺出味甘者，皆不治之证也，大法以救津液，壮水火为生。"

Definitions of Diabetic Kidney Disease

Typical descriptions of DKD that are consistent with modern understanding of DKD can be found in the classical literature. For example, in *Prescriptions and Expositions of Huangdi's Plain Questions* 黄帝素问宣明方论 published in the Jin dynasty (AD 1115–1234), *Xiao shen* 消肾 referred to symptoms of turbid urine caused by an unbalanced diet of sweet, pungent and hot foods. "或瘅或消中，善食而瘦。或消渴多虚，头面肿，小便数。或服甘辛热药过度，变成三消，上则消渴，中则消中，下则消肾，小便白膏也。"

In the book *Jing Yue Quan Shu* 景岳全书 from the Ming dynasty (AD 1368–1644), it mentions *Xia xiao* 下消 is a renal condition with symptoms of dark urine, turbid urine, dark complexion, and muscle wasting. As it is a renal disease, it is also named *Shen xiao* 肾消 (*Shen* means kidney in Chinese). 下消者，下焦病也。小便黄赤，为淋为浊，如膏如脂，面黑耳焦，日渐消瘦，其病在肾，故又名肾消也。

In another book also from the Ming dynasty, *Classified Classic* 类经, a similar description was recorded. *Shen xiao* 肾消 included symptoms of serious thirst relieved by continuous drinking, atrophy of the leg muscles and turbid urine. "若饮水多而小便多，名曰消渴；若饮食多，不甚渴，小便数而消瘦者，名曰消中；若渴而饮水不绝，腿消瘦而小便有脂液者，名曰肾消。"

In *Rewritten Treatise on Cold Damage* 重订通俗伤寒论 published in the Qing dynasty (AD 1644–1911), it states that if patients present with the syndrome of polydipsia, polyuria and abnormal urine including sweet urine and turbid urine, they were diagnosed as *Xia xiao* 下消. "如饮一溲一。色亦凝如白膏。味甜无臭者。三消症中之下消也。"

The aetiology of DKD was described in the book *Qi xiao liang fang* 奇效良方 from the Ming dynasty (AD 1368–1644). The main cause of disease was dietary irregularities, including overeating salty and fried foods, and alcoholism. In addition, disturbed emotions, other comorbid diseases, and misuse of mineral medicinals were also described as causes of DKD. The basic and common pathogenesis of disease was *yin* deficiency with internal heat. "三消之疾，本湿寒相搏，阴气极为燥热，阳气太甚，亦皆饮食服饵失宜，肠胃干涸，而气液不可宣平，或耗乱精神，过违其度。或因大病，阴气损而液衰，虚阳气悍，而燥热亦甚，或因久嗜咸物，恣食炙爆，饮酒过度。亦有年少服金石丸散，久积金石之毒，热结于胸中，下焦虚热益甚，因而肾水不能制，金石热燥甚于肾，故渴而引饮。若饮水多而小便多者，名曰消渴；若饮食多而不甚渴，小便数而消瘦者，名曰消中；若渴而饮水下不绝，肌消瘦而小便有脂膏者，名曰肾消。此三消者，其燥热同也。"

Chinese Herbal Medicine

Frequency of Treatment Citations by Dynasty

The first citation was found in the book *Bei ji qian jin yao fang* 备急千金药方 from the Tang dynasty (after AD 618) (Table 3.3). After Tang, the number of citations increased significantly in the Song and Jin dynasties. This is likely due to the increased number of publications during this period. There weren't any citations found in the Yuan dynasty which may be due to the short duration of this dynasty spanning less than 100 years. In addition, ethnicity changed from Han people to Mongolians and lifestyles shifted, which may be the reason for diabetes and its complications being absent from the medical literature in these dynasties.

Most of the citations were found in books published during the Ming and Qing dynasties. The increase in citations is likely due to an

Table 3.3.   Dynastic Distribution of Treatment Citations

Dynasty	No. of Treatment Citations
Before Tang Dynasty (before 618)	0
Tang and 5 Dynasties (618–960)	2 (3.4%)
Song and Jin Dynasties (960–1279)	17 (28.8%)
Yuan Dynasty (1271–1368)	0
Ming Dynasty (1368–1644)	26 (44.1%)
Qing Dynasty (1644–1911)	14 (23.7%)
Ming Guo/Republic of China (1912–1949)	0
Total	**59 (100%)**

increased number of publications including the official medical encyclopaedia, during the period. For example, the book that recorded the most citations was *Pu ji fang* 普济方, which was the most comprehensive pharmacopoeia published by the Chinese Government in the Ming dynasty.

Treatment with Chinese Herbal Medicine

Chinese herbal medicine (CHM) was used in all of the 59 citations. Other CM treatments, such as acupuncture and moxibustion, were not found in included citations. Based on the coding scores, included citations were pooled into two groups, that is, 'possible DKD' and 'most likely DKD'. There were 59 citations in the possible DKD pool and, out of the 59 citations, 22 were considered to be most likely DKD. Data analysis was performed and compared within these two different pools (Fig. 3.2).

Most Frequent Formulae in Possible Diabetic Kidney Disease Citations

Of the 59 possible DKD citations, 33 unique formulae consisting of 82 herbs were found. The formulae were diverse and about half were cited only once and the other half cited between two and four times.

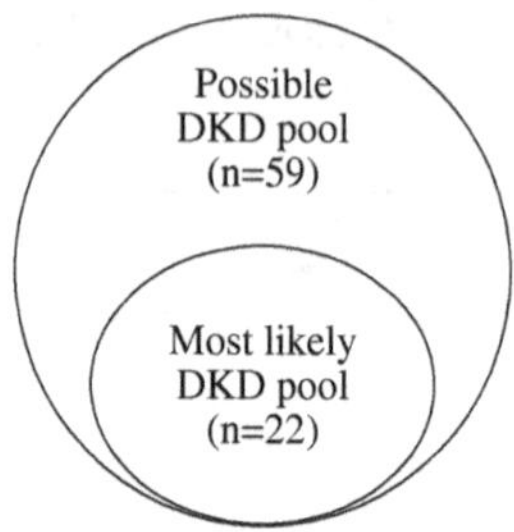

Fig. 3.2. Relationship between possible diabetic kidney disease (DKD) and most likely DKD citations.

The most frequent formulae were cited four times each and included *Hui xiang san* 茴香散, *Liu wei di huang wan* 六味地黄丸 and *Ba wei wan* 八味丸 (Table 3.4).

Hui xiang san 茴香散 for the treatment of DKD was recorded in the Pharmacopeia entries of the Ming and Qing dynasties, including the famous *Ben Cao Gang Mu* 本草纲目. *Hui xiang san* 茴香散 was cited for patients with a history of diabetes and symptoms of thirst and turbid urine (proteinuria). The ingredients of *Hui xiang san* 茴香散 were simple and included *xiao hui xiang* 小茴香 and *chuan lian zi* 川楝子. The formula targets the Kidney and Liver with the function of tonifying Kidney and regulating *qi*.

The formulae *Liu wei di huang wan* 六味地黄丸 and *Ba wei wan* 八味丸 have similar herbs and similar functions to tonify the Kidney. *Liu* and *Ba* are the number six and number eight in Chinese, which states the number of ingredients in the formulae. *Ba wei wan* 八味丸 was first recorded in the Han dynasty in the book *Jin Gui Yao Lue* 金匮要略, in which it was named *Cui's ba wei wan* 崔氏八味丸 and also named *Ba wei shen qi wan* 八味肾气丸. It contains *fu zi* 附子, *gui zhi* 桂枝, *di huang* 地黄, *shan zhu yu* 山茱萸, *ze xie* 泽泻, *mu dan pi* 牡丹皮, *shan yao* 山药, and *fu ling* 茯苓. *Liu wei di huang wan* 六味地黄丸 was created by doctor *Qian yi* 钱乙 in the Song dynasty, and derived from *Ba wei wan* 八味丸 by removing two warm-tonifying herbs. The distinct herbs in these two formulae are *fu zi* 附子 and *gui zhi* 桂枝, which distinguish the tonifying *yang* effect of *Ba wei wan*

Table 3.4.   Most Frequent Formulae in Possible Diabetic Kidney Disease Citations

Formula Name	Herb Ingredients	No. of Citations
Hui xiang san 茴香散	*Xiao hui xiang* 小茴香, *chuan lian zi* 川楝子	4
Ba wei wan 八味丸	*Fu zi* 附子, *gui zhi* 桂枝, *di huang* 地黄, *shan zhu yu* 山茱萸, *ze xie* 泽泻, *mu dan pi* 牡丹皮, *shan yao* 山药, *fu ling* 茯苓	4
Liu wei di huang wan 六味地黄丸	*Di huang* 地黄, *shan zhu yu* 山茱萸, *ze xie* 泽泻, *mu dan pi* 牡丹皮, *shan yao* 山药, *fu ling* 茯苓	4
Shen li tang / Ci shi tang 肾沥汤/磁石汤	*Ci shi* 磁石, *huang qi* 黄芪, *ren shen* 人参, *wu wei zi* 五味子, *du zhong* 杜仲, *shu di huang* 熟地黄, *yang shen* 羊肾	3
Sao si tang/Yuan can jian tang 缲丝汤/原蚕茧汤	*Jian si* 茧丝/*Can jian* 蚕茧	3
Tu si zi san 菟丝子散	*Tu si zi* 菟丝子, *pu huang* 蒲黄, *ci shi* 磁石, *huang lian* 黄连, *rou cong rong* 肉苁蓉, *wu wei zi* 五味子, *ji nei jing* 鸡内金	3

Note: The use of some herbs may be restricted in some countries; readers are advised to comply with relevant regulations.

八味丸 from the nourishing *yin* effect of *Liu wei di huang wan* 六味地黄丸. Both of the formulae were used for diabetes with thirst, polyuria, frequent urination and turbid urine.

Another commonly used formula was *Sao si tang* 缲丝汤, also called Reeling Silk Decoction. It is a single herb formula containing *jian si* 茧丝 (silk cocoon or silk floss). All four citations of *Sao si tang* 缲丝汤 were from the Ming dynasty and it was used for turbid urine, polydipsia and excessive appetite with muscle atrophy. The citations also mentioned that salty foods should be avoided during treatment. Modern research indicates that the main active compounds of silk cocoon and silkworm can decrease urine albumin excretion and reduce blood glucose levels in patients with type 2 diabetes.[6]

Shen li tang 肾沥汤 and *Ci shi tang* 磁石汤 are two formulae with identical ingredients. The formula contains six commonly used herbs combined with lamb kidney (Table 3.4). It is used to treat patients presenting with turbid urine and weight loss with Kidney deficiency.

Tu si zi san 菟丝子散 is a formula of herbal mixed powder which was recorded for the treatment of patients with polyuria and turbid urine in the Song and Ming dynasties. This formula should be used before meals to warm the Kidney.

Most Frequent Herbs in Possible Diabetic Kidney Disease Citations

In the possible DKD citations, 82 unique herbs were mentioned. The frequencies of herbs ranged from one to 24 and most (85%) were mentioned in less than ten citations. Therefore, herbs which were cited more than ten times were regarded as high frequency herbs. As a result, 12 herbs had a high frequency and the top three herbs were *fu ling* 茯苓, *ren shen* 人参, and *shu di huang* 熟地黄 (Table 3.5).

Table 3.5. Most Frequent Herbs in Possible Diabetic Kidney Disease Citations

Herb Name	Scientific Name	No. of Citations
Fu ling 茯苓	*Poria cocos* (Schw.) Wolf	24
Ren shen 人参	*Panax ginseng* C. A. Mey.	20
Shu di huang 熟地黄	*Rehmannia glutinosa* Libosch.	20
Wu wei zi 五味子	*Schisandra chinensis* (Turcz.) Baill.	18
Ze xie 泽泻	*Alisma orientalis* (Sam.) Juzep.	18
Huang lian 黄连	*Coptis spp.*	14
Shan yao 山药	*Dioscorea opposita* Thunb.	14
Shan zhu yu 山茱萸	*Cornus officinalis* Sieb. et Zucc.	13
Mu dan pi 牡丹皮	*Paeonia suffruticosa* Andr.	11
Mu li 牡蛎	*Ostrea spp.*	11
Ji nei jin 鸡内金	*Gallus gallus domesticus* Brisson	10
Tian hua fen 天花粉	*Trichosanthes spp.*	10

Note: The use of some herbs may be restricted in some countries; readers are advised to comply with relevant regulations.

The high frequency herbs aligned with the ingredients of *Liu wei di huang wan* 六味地黄丸 and similar formulae that tonify the Kidney. The high frequency herbs can be categorised into four main groups, including tonics and replenishing herbs, astringents, digestants and heat-clearing medicinals. These herb categories reflect the CM theory that DKD is due to deficiency, stagnation and/or heat.

Most Frequent Formulae in Most Likely Diabetic Kidney Disease Citations

Twenty-two citations were sub grouped from the possible DKD pool because the citation described conditions that were most likely DKD. They included a full description of diabetes progression, diabetes symptoms and kidney disorder. The descriptions indicated they were consistent with DKD as it is understood today.

In the 22 most likely DKD citations, 13 unique formulae with 59 herbs were mentioned. Frequencies of formulae ranged from one to three and only six formulae were cited more than once (Table 3.6). The most frequent formulae were *Sao si tang/Yuan can jian tang* 缫丝汤/原蚕茧汤 and *Liu wei di huang wan* 六味地黄丸.

The other formulae used in multiple citations were *Gu ben wan* 固本丸, *Hua cong rong wan* 花苁蓉丸, *Tian hua wan* 天花丸, and *Zhi bo ba wei wan* 知柏八味丸. These formulae were all used for long-term diabetes with severe thirst, polyuria and turbid urine, except for *Hua cong rong wan* 花苁蓉丸 which was used for diabetes and lower limb oedema.

Most Frequent Herbs in Most Likely Diabetic Kidney Disease Citations

In the most likely DKD citations, 59 unique herbs were found. The frequencies of herbs ranged from one to 12. Nine herbs were considered to be high frequency because they were reported in five or more citations (Table 3.7). The top three herbs were *fu ling* 茯苓, *ze xie* 泽泻, and *shu di huang* 熟地黄.

Table 3.6. Most Frequent Formulae in Most Likely Diabetic Kidney Disease Citations

Formula Name	Herb Ingredients	No. of Citations
Sao si tang/Yuan can jian tang 缫丝汤/原蚕茧汤	*Jian si* 茧丝/*Can jian* 蚕茧	3
Liu wei di huang wan 六味地黄丸	*Di huang* 地黄, *shan zhu yu* 山茱萸, *ze xie* 泽泻, *mu dan pi* 牡丹皮, *shan yao* 山药, *fu ling* 茯苓	3
Ba wei wan 八味丸	*Fu zi* 附子, *gui zhi* 桂枝, *di huang* 地黄, *shan zhu yu* 山茱萸, *ze xie* 泽泻, *mu dan pi* 牡丹皮, *shan yao* 山药, *fu ling* 茯苓	2
Gu ben wan 固本丸	*Sheng di huang* 生地黄, *shu di huang* 熟地黄, *tian dong* 天冬, *mai dong* 麦冬	2
Hua cong rong wan 花苁蓉丸	*Hua cong rong* 花苁蓉, *ze xie* 泽泻, *wu wei zi* 五味子, *ba ji tian* 巴戟天, *di gu pi* 地骨皮, *gua lou* 瓜蒌, *ci shi* 磁石, *ren shen* 人参, *chi shi zhi* 赤石脂, *gan jiang* 干姜, *yu yu liang* 禹余粮, *shan piao xiao* 桑螵蛸, mang xiao 芒硝	2
Tian hua wan 天花丸	*Tian hua fen* 天花粉, *fu ling* 茯苓, *mu li* 牡蛎, *zhi mu* 知母, *tie fen* 铁粉, *ku shen* 苦参, *zhu sha* 朱砂, *bai bian dou* 白扁豆, *huang lian* 黄连, *lu hui* 芦荟, *jin yin bo* 金银箔	2
Zhi bo ba wei wan 知柏八味丸	*Zhi mu* 知母, *huang bai* 黄柏, *shu di huang* 熟地黄, *shan zhu yu* 山茱萸, *ze xie* 泽泻, *mu dan pi* 牡丹皮, *shan yao* 山药, *fu ling* 茯苓	2

Note: The use of some herbs may be restricted in some countries; readers are advised to comply with relevant regulations.

The most frequent herbs in the most likely DKD citations included the ingredients of *Liu wei di huang wan* 六味地黄丸 and tonifying herbs such as *ren shen* 人参 and heat-clearing herbs such as *zhi mu* 知母.

Table 3.7. Most Frequent Herbs in Most Likely Diabetic Kidney Disease Citations

Herb Name	Scientific Name	No. of Citations
Fu ling 茯苓	*Poria cocos* (Schw.) Wolf	12
Ze xie 泽泻	*Alisma orientalis* (Sam.) Juzep.	12
Shu di huang 熟地黄	*Rehmannia glutinosa* Libosch.	11
Shan zhu yu 山茱萸	*Cornus officinalis* Sieb. et Zucc.	9
Mu dan pi 牡丹皮	*Paeonia suffruticosa* Andr.	8
Shan yao 山药	*Dioscorea opposita* Thunb.	8
Ren shen 人参	*Panax ginseng* C. A. Mey.	6
Tian hua fen 天花粉	*Trichosanthes spp.*	5
Zhi mu 知母	*Anemarrhena asphodeloides* Bge.	5

Note: The use of some herbs may be restricted in some countries; readers are advised to comply with relevant regulations.

Most Frequent Formulae and Herbs in Citations Describing Specific Symptoms

The most common symptom of DKD in the classical literature citations was turbid urine referred to in 57 citations (96.6%). Frequent urination and polyuria with or without profuse drinking was described in 37 citations (62.7%). Typical disorders of diabetes such as thirst and weight loss were recorded in a similar number of citations (19 and 17, respectively). Lower limb oedema was less commonly reported and was only mentioned in three citations. Other symptoms of diabetes, including increased appetite and sweet urine were only found in one citation each. Most of the symptoms described in the included citations are symptoms presenting at the early stage of DKD. Frequency analyses were conducted based on individual symptoms. Of the citations that mentioned specific symptoms, the same high frequency formulae and herbs found in the overall pool of possible DKD citations were used (Table 3.4 and Table 3.5). Except for *huang qi* 黄芪, that was frequently reported in citations mentioning turbid urine or weight loss.

Selected Quotes

Quotes of typical medical cases of treatments for possible DKD or most likely DKD were selected and translated. In the book *Sun Wen Yuan's Medical Records* 孙文垣医案 written in the Ming and Qing dynasties, there is a record of a patient in his 50s, who was addicted to alcohol for years, suffered from frequent urination more than 20 times per night for half a year and his urine became sweet and turbid. Gradually, he lost his appetite and became weak. Dr. *Sun* prescribed a pill formula containing *shu di huang, lu jiao shuang, shan zhu yu, sang piao xiao, lu xiao jiao, ren shen, fu ling, gou qi zi, yuan zhi, tu si zi, shan yao, yi zhi ren, fu zi, gui zhi* and honey, and told the patient to take the pills in the morning and evening with weak brine. The patient recovered before finishing all the prescribed pills. "一书办下消，一书办年过五十，糟酒纵欲无惮，忽患下消之症，一日夜小便二十余度，清白而长，味且甜，少顷凝结如脂，色有油光。治半年不验，腰膝以下皆软弱，载身不起，饮食减半，神色大瘁。脉之六部大而无力。书云：脉至而从，按之不鼓，诸阳皆然，法当温补下焦。以熟地黄六两为君，鹿角霜、山茱萸各四两，桑螵蛸、鹿角胶、人参、白茯苓、枸杞子、远志、菟丝子、怀山药各三两为臣，益智仁一两为佐，大附子、桂心各七钱为使，炼蜜为丸，梧桐子大，每早晚淡盐汤送下七八十丸，不终剂而愈。"《孙文亘医案 · 卷二 · 三吴治验》(书办：明、清时期，府、州、县署名房书吏的通称。掌管文书，核拟稿件，嗣后用为掌案书吏的专称)

Another typical case was recorded in the book *Medical Records for Clinical Practice Guidance* 临证指南医案. A patient felt thirsty and drank a lot of water, and always felt hungry, with turbid urine. The doctor diagnosed *Shen xiao* 肾消, and considered the patient to have more than a minor illness, and prescribed a formula containing *shu di huang, shan zhu yu, shan yao, fu ling, niu xi, che qian zi.* "杨（二六） 渴饮频饥。溲溺浑浊。此属肾消。阴精内耗。阳气上燔。舌碎绛赤。乃阴不上承。非客热宜此。乃脏液无存。岂是平常小恙。熟地，萸肉，山药，茯神，牛膝，车前子。"《临证指南医案 · 卷六 · 三消》

Acupuncture and Related Therapies

Four citations recorded acupuncture and moxibustion from the Song, Ming and Qing dynasties. However, none of them were included, because they were judged as not likely to be DKD.

Classical Literature in Perspective

Classical literature written over 2,500 years provides important information that continues to guide modern clinical practice. Search terms, X*ia xiao* 下消, S*hen xiao* 肾消, X*iao shen* 消肾, described conditions very similar to diabetes and its complications although there were no specific terms used in the classical literature that directly corresponded to DKD in modern language. Therefore possible treatments from classical literature were based on the common symptomatic appearance of DKD and diabetic symptoms. All three search terms located a similar number of citations both at the initial search and after a judgement regarding the likelihood of being DKD was applied. Therefore, this confirmed that one term was not more like a modern definition of DKD than the others.

Citations were distributed throughout dynastic China from the Tang and 5 dynasties to the Qing dynasty. Most citations were found in books written and published in the Ming dynasty (AD 1369–1644) and Qing dynasty (AD 1645–1911). DKD was reported in classical literature citations but the number of citations was small. This may be due to the limited number of search terms. While the three search terms had reasonable specificity to identify citations which were consistent with DKD, they may not have been broad enough to capture all possible DKD citations. DKD citations were also difficult to identify because DKD diagnosis is currently based on laboratory testing, which was not available in ancient times. Therefore finding descriptions of DKD based on symptoms was difficult and required careful inspection of the citation details.

All included DKD citations recorded the treatments for early stage DKD. The common formulae and herbs were similar between the possible and most likely pools. The most common formulae *Liu wei di huang wan* 六味地黄丸 and *Ba wei wan* 八味丸 are still widely used today. These formulae and their modified formulae, such as *Shen qi di huang wan* 参芪地黄丸, *Qi ju di huang wang* 杞菊地黄丸, and *Ji sheng shen qi wan* 济生肾气丸, are recommended in the modern CM clinical guidelines for DKD.[7] This suggests that the traditional knowledge has informed modern CM practice.

The herbs included in the formula were often tonics, astringents, digestants and heat-clearing herbs. These results closely correspond to the herbs commonly used for DKD today. Furthermore, results of herbal analysis based on individual symptoms show *huang qi* 黄芪 was commonly used for the treatment of turbid urine. The results of a systematic review that assessed the effectiveness of *huang qi* 黄芪 products showed that this herb reduced urine albumin excretion in diabetic nephropathy paitients.[8]

There are some differences between ancient treatments of DKD and treatments today. For example, *Jian si* 茧丝 has been researched for its anti-diabetic and anti-albuminuria in pre-clinical studies but it is not commonly used in clinical practice.[6] Additionally, some of the formulae contained mineral compounds and these should be used with caution in clinical practice.

Apart from citations that used CHM treatment, there were few relevant citations that used acupuncture or other CM therapies.

Overall, the results show that ancient treatments of DKD are similar to modern treatments. Formula and herbs have been continually and consistently used over thousands of years to treat DKD symptoms.

References

1. Hu R, ed. (2000) Zhong Hua Yi Dian "Encyclopaedia of Traditional Chinese Medicine." 4 ed., Changsha: Hunan Electronic and Audio-Visual Publishing House.
2. May BH, Lu CJ, Xue CCL. (2012) Collections of traditional Chinese medical literature as resources for systematic searches. *J Altern Complement Med* **18**(12): 1101–1107.

3. May BH, Lu YB, Lu CJ, Zhang AL, *et al.* (2013) Systematic assessment of the representativeness of published collections of the traditional literature on Chinese Medicine. *J Altern Complement Med* **19**(5): 403–409.
4. Zhang L, Li Y, Guo X, May BH, *et al.* (2014) Text mining of the classical medical literature for medicines that show potential in diabetic nephropathy. *Evid Based Complement Alternat Med*, Article ID 189125.
5. 国家中医药管理局医政司. 22 个专业　95 个病种中医诊疗方案. 北京. 2010: 167–192.
6. Zhang L, Zhang La, Li Y, Guo X, Liu X. (2015) Biotransformation effect of Bombyx Mori L. may play an important role in treating diabetic nephropathy. *Chin J Integr Med* 2015: 1–8.
7. 中华中医药学会糖尿病分会. 糖尿病肾脏疾病中医诊疗标准. 世界中西医结合杂志. 2011. **6**(6): 548–552.
8. Li M, Wang W, Xue J, Gu Y, Lin S. (2011) Meta-analysis of the clinical value of Astragalus membranaceus in diabetic nephropathy. *J Ethnopharmacol* **133**(2): 412–419.

4

Methods for Evaluating Clinical Evidence

OVERVIEW

This chapter describes the methods used to identify and evaluate a range of Chinese medicine interventions for diabetic kidney disease in clinical studies. Studies identified through a comprehensive search were assessed against eligibility criteria. A review of the methodological quality of the studies was undertaken using standardised methods. Results from included studies were evaluated to provide an estimate of the effects of a range of Chinese medicine therapies.

Introduction

The use of Chinese medicine (CM) for diabetic kidney disease (DKD) has been well described in the contemporary literature. Clinical trials and systematic reviews have been conducted to evaluate the efficacy and safety of CM treatments for DKD.

This chapter describes the methods for examining CM interventions for DKD in clinical studies. CM interventions have been categorised as follows:

- Chinese herbal medicine (CHM)(Chapter 5)
- Acupuncture and related therapies (Chapter 7)
- Other CM therapies (Chapter 8)
- Combination CM therapies (Chapter 9).

References to clinical trials were obtained and assessed by an expert group including the authors, co-authors and advisory panel.

Randomised controlled trials (RCTs), non-randomised controlled clinical trials (CCTs) and non-controlled studies were evaluated in detail. CCTs were evaluated using the same approach as RCTs, and have been described separately. Evidence from non-controlled studies is more difficult to evaluate, therefore the approach was taken to describe the characteristics of the study, details of the intervention and any adverse events. References to the included studies can be found at the end of chapters 5, 7, 8, and 9. References are indicated by a letter followed by a number. Studies of CHM are indicated by an 'H' (e.g. H1), studies of acupuncture and related therapies indicated by an 'A' (e.g. A1), studies of other CM therapies indicated by an 'O' (e.g. O1), and studies of combinations of CM therapies indicated by a 'C' (e.g. C1).

Search Strategy

Evidence was searched in English and Chinese language databases and the methods followed the Cochrane Handbook of Systematic Reviews.[1] English-language databases included PubMed, Excerpta Medica Database (Embase), Cumulative Index of Nursing and Allied Health Literature (CINAHL), Cochrane Central Register of Controlled Trials (CENTRAL), including the Cochrane Library, and Allied and Complementary Medicine Database (AMED); and Chinese-language databases included China BioMedical Literature (CBM), China National Knowledge Infrastructure (CNKI), Chonqing VIP (CQVIP) and Wanfang. Databases were searched from inception to April 2015. No restrictions were applied. Search terms were mapped to controlled vocabulary (where applicable) in addition to being searched as keywords.

To conduct a comprehensive search of the literature, searches were run according to the study design (reviews, controlled trials, non-controlled studies). This was done for each of the three intervention types (CHM, acupuncture and related therapies, and other CM therapies) resulting in nine searches in each of the nine databases:

1. CHM reviews
2. CHM controlled trials (randomised and non-randomised)

3. CHM non-controlled studies
4. Acupuncture & related therapies reviews
5. Acupuncture & related therapies controlled trials (randomised and non-randomised)
6. Acupuncture & related therapies non-controlled studies
7. Other CM therapies reviews
8. Other CM therapies controlled trials (randomised and non-randomised)
9. Other CM therapies non-controlled studies.

Studies of combination CM therapies were identified through the above searches. In addition to electronic databases, reference lists of systematic reviews and included studies were searched for additional publications. Clinical trial registries were searched to identify clinical trials which were ongoing or completed, and where required, trial investigators were contacted to obtain data. The searched trial registries included the Australian New Zealand Clinical Trial Registry (ANZCTR), the Chinese Clinical Trial Registry (ChiCTR), the European Union Clinical Trials Register (EU-CTR), and the U.S.A. National Institutes of Health registry (ClinicalTrials.gov).

Inclusion Criteria

- Participants: Adults with diabetes mellitus (either type 1 or type 2) complicated by stage 1–3 (i.e early stage) DKD with microalbuminuria.[2] Microalbuminuria is indicated by urine albumin-creatinine ratio (ACR) between 30 and 300 mg/g or urine albumin excretion rate (AER) between 30 and 300 mg/24h or between 20 to 200 μg/min in timed collection.[3]
- Interventions: CHM, acupuncture and related therapies, or other CM therapies. Integrative medicine, such as CHM plus pharmacotherapy, was also investigated (see Table 4.1)
- Comparators: Placebo, or conventional therapies (CT) recommended in guidelines such as blood glucose, blood pressure, and blood lipid control, lifestyle advice including diet modification, and exercise.[3,4]

Table 4.1. Chinese Medicine Interventions Included in Clinical Evidence Evaluation

Category	Intervention
Chinese herbal medicines (CHM)	Oral CHM, CHM enema
Acupuncture and related therapies	Acupuncture, moxibustion, point application therapy
Other Chinese medicine therapies	*Tai chi* 太极, Chinese diet therapy
Combination Chinese medicine therapies	Combination therapies are defined as two or more Chinese medicine interventions from different categories administered together e.g. CHM plus acupuncture

- Outcome measures: Studies reported at least one of the pre-specified outcome measures (Table 4.2).

Exclusion Criteria

- Patients receiving renal replacement therapy (dialysis or transplant).
- Non-DKD.
- Studies which lack a standard CM treatment. For example studies that prescribe individualised treatments based on CM syndromes such as *yin* deficiency or *qi* deficiency.
- Control not routinely recommended for DKD in international clinical practice guidelines or no treatment control.
- Control therapies include any type of CM therapies.
- Integrative medicine studies that used different therapies in the intervention groups compared to the control group.

Outcomes

Pre-specified outcomes of effect included known measures in DKD research including mortality, events indicating progression of disease, change in kidney function, markers of kidney damage, quality of life, indicators of risk factor control, health care costs and adverse events.

Table 4.2. Pre-specified Outcomes

Outcome Category	Outcome Measures	Scoring
	PRIMARY OUTCOMES	
Mortality	All-cause mortality	Number of participants; lower is better

Events indicating progression	1. Progression to end-stage kidney/renal disease (ESRD)
	2. Doubling of serum creatinine (SCr) from baseline
	3. Percentage decline in glomerular filtration rate (GFR) or estimated GFR (eGFR): (30%, 40% or 50%)
	4. Change in chronic kidney disease (CKD) stage
	5. Progression or regression of albuminuria
	   a. micro-to-macro
	   b. micro-to-normo
		1. Number of participants; lower is better
		2. Number of participants; lower is better
		3. Number of participants; lower is better
		4. Number of participants; lower stage is better
		5. Number of participants
		   a. Lower is better
		   b. Higher is better

Change in kidney function	1. GFR or eGFR 2. SCr concentration 3. Creatinine clearance (CrCl)	1. Normal range ≥ 90 mL/min/1.73 cm^2 2. Female; 0.50–1.10 mg/dL; male 0.70 ~ 1.30 mg/dL 3. Normal range ≥ 90 mL/min

Markers of kidney damage	1. Proteinuria
	2. Albumin excretion rate (AER)
	3. Urine albumin-creatinine ratio (ACR)
	4. Urine protein creatinine ratio (PCR)
		1. Normal range < 100 mg/24h
		2. Normal range < 20 µg/min or <30 mg/24h
		   a. Micro: 30 ~ 300 mg/24h or 20 ~ 200 µg/min
		   b. Macro: >300 mg/24h or >200 µg/min
		3. Normal range < 3.4 mg/mmol or <30 mg/g
		   a. Micro: 3.4 ~ 34 mg/mmol or 30 ~ 300 mg/g
		   b. Macro: >34 mg/mmol or >300 mg/g
		4. Normal range < 0.2 mg/mg

(Continued)

Table 4.2. (*Continued*)

Outcome Category	Outcome Measures	Scoring
SECONDARY OUTCOMES		
Mortality	Cardiovascular mortality	Number of participants; lower is better
Hospitalisation	All cause hospitalisation	Number of participants; lower is better
Quality of life	Any validated measure	Varies based on the measure used
Indicators of risk factor control	1. Fasting blood glucose (FBG) 2. Hemoglobin A1c (HbA1c) 3. Systolic blood pressure (SBP) 4. Diastolic blood pressure (DBP) 5. Total cholesterol 6. LDL cholesterol 7. HDL cholesterol 8. Triglycerides 9. Serum urine acid level	1. Normal range 3.9 ~ 5.5 mmol/L or 70 ~ 99 mg/dL 2. Normal range 20 ~ 38 mmol/mol or 4 ~ 5.6% 3. Normal range 90 ~ 140 mmHg 4. Normal range 60 ~ 90 mmHg 5. Desirable < 200 mg/dL 6. Optimal < 100 mg/dL 7. Female: <50 mg/dL; Male: <40 mg/dL 8. Normal range ≤ 250 mg/dL or 2.82 mmol/L 9. Normal range 3 ~ 7 mg/dL or 178 ~ 416 μmol/L
Healthcare costs	Total health care costs	
Adverse Events	Number and type of adverse events	

Note: Changes in kidney function may vary depending on age, gender and race. The normal values referenced in this table are used as a guide only and may not be accurate depending on patient variables.

Abbreviations: AER, albumin excretion rate; ACR, urine albumin creatinine ratio; CKD, chronic kidney disease; CrCl creatinine clearance; DBP, diastolic blood pressure; eGFR, estimated glomerular filtration rate; ESRD, end-stage renal disease; FBG; Fasting blood glucose; GFR, glomerular filtration rate; HbA1c, haemoglobin A1c; HDL, high-density lipoprotein; LDL, low-density lipoprotein; PCR, protein creatinine ratio; SBP, systolic blood pressure; SCr, serum creatinine.

These outcomes were gathered from clinical practice guidelines and then selected according to their rated importance by the nephrology expert advisory panel of this monograph.[3–5] The pre-specified outcomes included both clinical outcomes and surrogate biomedical markers related to DKD severity, as well as patient-centred outcomes such as quality of life. The outcomes and measurements are specified in Table 4.2.

Outcome data measured at the end of treatment and at the end of follow-up were included in meta-analysis. For the outcomes of mortality, events indicating progression, hospitalisation and adverse events, the numbers of events in each group were counted and analysed as dichotomous data. For other biomedical measures, such as quality of life and health care cost, continuous outcome data were extracted and analysed by comparing the between group differences.

Risk of Bias Assessment

Risk of bias was assessed for RCTs using the Cochrane Collaboration tool.[1] In clinical trials, bias can be categorised as selection bias, performance bias, detection bias, attrition bias, and reporting bias. Each domain was assessed to determine whether the bias was at low, high, or unclear risk. Low risk of bias indicated that bias was unlikely, high risk indicated plausible bias that seriously weakened confidence in the results and unclear bias indicated lack of information or uncertainty over potential bias and raised some doubt about the results. Risk of bias assessment was verified by two people and disagreement was resolved by discussion or consultation with a third person.

Risk of bias was categorised using the following six domains:

- Sequence generation: the method used to generate the allocation sequence was given in sufficient detail to allow an assessment of whether it should produce comparable groups. Low risk of bias referred to a random number table or computer random generator. High risk of bias included studies that described a non-random sequence generation, such as odd or even date of birth or date of admission.
- Allocation concealment: the method used to conceal the allocation sequence was given in enough detail to determine whether intervention allocations could have been foreseen before or during

enrolment. Low risk of bias included central randomisation or sealed envelopes and high risk of bias included open random sequence, date of birth, etc.

- Blinding of participants and personnel: measures used to describe if the study participants and personnel were blinded to the intervention received. In addition, information relating to whether the blinding was effective was also assessed. Studies that ensured blinding of participants and personnel were at low risk of bias. If the study was not blinded or incompletely blinded, it was deemed at high risk of bias.
- Blinding of outcome assessors: measures used to describe if the outcome assessors were blinded to knowledge of which intervention a participant received. Additional assessment for blinding efficacy was performed as per the above dot point.
- Incomplete outcome data: completeness of outcome data for each main outcome, including drop outs, exclusions from the analysis with numbers missing in each group and reasons for drop out or exclusions. Studies with low risk of bias included all outcome data or, if there was missing data, these were unlikely to be related to the true outcome or were balanced between groups. Studies at high risk of bias had unexplained missing data.
- Selective reporting: the study protocol was available and the pre-specified outcomes were included in the report. Studies with a published protocol and included all pre-specified outcomes in their report were at low risk of bias. Studies at high risk of bias were those that did not include all pre-specified outcomes or reported at least some of them incompletely.

Statistical Analyses

Frequencies of CM syndromes, CHM formulae, herbs and acupuncture points reported in included studies are presented using descriptive statistics. CM syndromes reported in two or more studies are presented. The 10 most frequently reported CHM formulae and 20 most frequently reported herbs are presented when used in at least two studies, although for CHM formulae this was not always possible. Where data was limited, reports of single CM syndromes or acupuncture points are provided as a guide for the reader.

Definitions of statistical tests and results are described in the glossary. Dichotomous data are reported as a risk ratio (RR) with 95% confidence intervals (CI), and continuous data are reported as mean difference (MD) with 95% CI. For all pooled analyses, estimates of heterogeneity are reported with RR or MD and 95% CI. Formal tests for heterogeneity were conducted using the I^2 statistic. An I^2 score greater than 50% was considered to indicate substantial heterogeneity.[1] Where possible and appropriate, planned subgroup analyses included duration of treatment, CM formula, comparator type, washout for angiotensin-converting enzyme inhibitor (ACEI) or angiotensin receptor blockers (ARB), and baseline kidney function. Sensitivity analyses were undertaken to explore potential sources of heterogeneity, based on low risk of bias for sequence generation. Available case analysis with a random effects model was used in all analyses. The random effects model was used to take into account the clinical heterogeneity likely to be encountered within and between included studies, and the variation in treatment effects between included studies.

Assessment Using Grading of Recommendations Assessment, Development and Evaluation (GRADE)

The Grading of Recommendations Assessment, Development and Evaluation (GRADE) approach was used.[6] The GRADE approach summarises and rates the quality of evidence in systematic reviews using a structured process for presenting evidence summaries. The results are presented in summary of findings tables. The results provide an important overview for DKD outcomes.

A panel of experts was established to evaluate the quality of evidence. The panel included the systematic review team, CM practitioners, integrative medicine experts, research methodologists, and conventional medicine physicians. The experts were asked to rate the clinical importance of key interventions from CHM, acupuncture therapies and other CM therapies, as well as comparators and outcomes.

Results were collated and, based on the rating scores and subsequent discussion, a consensus on the content for the summary of findings tables was achieved.

The quality of evidence for each outcome was rated according to five factors outlined in the GRADE approach:

- Limitations in study design (risk of bias),
- Inconsistency of results (unexplained heterogeneity),
- Indirectness of evidence (interventions, populations and outcomes important to the patients with the condition),
- Imprecision (uncertainty about the results), and
- Publication bias (selective publication of studies).

These five factors are additive and a reduction in more than one factor will reduce the quality of the evidence for that outcome. The GRADE approach also includes three domains that can be rated up, including large magnitude of an effect, dose-response gradient and effect of plausible residual confounding. However, these three domains more commonly relate to observational studies including cohort, case-control, before-after, time series studies, etc. GRADE summaries in this monograph only included RCTs; therefore these three domains for rating up were not assessed.

Treatment recommendations can also be assessed using the GRADE approach but, due to the diverse nature of CM practice, treatment recommendations were not included with the summary of findings. Therefore, the reader should interpret the evidence with reference to their local practice environment. It should also be noted that the GRADE approach requires judgments about the quality of evidence and some subjective assessment. However, the experience of the panel members suggests the judgments are reliable and transparent representations of the quality of evidence.

The GRADE levels of evidence are grouped into four categories:

1) High quality evidence: We are very confident that the true effect lies close to that of the estimate of the effect.

2) Moderate quality evidence: We are moderately confident in the effect estimate: The true effect is likely to be close to the estimate of the effect, but there is a possibility that it is substantially different.

3) Low quality evidence: Our confidence in the effect estimate is limited: The true effect may be substantially different from the estimate of the effect.

4) Very low quality evidence: We have very little confidence in the effect estimate: The true effect is likely to be substantially different from the estimate of effect.

References

1. Higgins J, Green S. (eds.) (2011) Cochrane Handbook for Systematic Reviews of Interventions Version 5.1.0 (The Cochrane Collaboration). Retrieved from http://www.cochrane-handbook.org

2. Mogensen CE, Christensen CK, Vittinghus E. (1983) The stages in diabetic renal disease. With emphasis on the stage of incipient diabetic nephropathy. *Diabetes* **32**(Suppl 2): 64–78.

3. KDOQI Clinical practice guidelines and clinical practice recommendations for diabetes and chronic kidney disease. (2007) *Am J Kidney Dis* **49**(Suppl 2): S12–154.

4. National Kidney Foundation. (2012) KDOQI Clinical Practice Guideline for Diabetes and CKD: 2012 update. *Am J Kidney Dis* **60**(5): 850–886.

5. American Diabetes Association. (2015) Microvascular complications and foot care. *Diabetes Care* **38**(Suppl 1): S58–S66.

6. Schunemann H, Brozek J, Guyatt G, Oxman A. (eds.) (2013) GRADE handbook for grading quality of evidence and strength of recommendations (The GRADE Working Group). Retrieved from http://www.guidelinedevelopment.org/handbook/

5

Clinical Evidence for Chinese Herbal Medicine

OVERVIEW

This chapter provides a synopsis of the clinical studies on Chinese herbal medicine (CHM) for early diabetic kidney disease (DKD). Previous systematic reviews are qualitatively described. Randomised controlled trials and non-randomised controlled clinical trials are systematically reviewed and meta-analyses are applied to evaluate the efficacy and safety of CHM for DKD. In addition, non-controlled studies have seen identified as supplementary. The non-controlled studies provide an overview of the interventions used and safety data of CHM for DKD.

Introduction

Chinese herbal medicine (CHM) in the management of diabetic kidney disease (DKD) has been evaluated in numerous clinical studies. CHM interventions typically employ multi-herb ingredient formulae as well as single-herb formulae which were documented in ancient Chinese medicine (CM) literature or developed according to CM theory by contemporary clinical physicians. CHMs are often given orally with a variety of preparation types, including liquid extractions, powder capsules, pills, and granules. The efficacy and safety of CHMs for the management of DKD patients with microalbuminuria were assessed and results presented in this chapter.

Previous Systematic Reviews

Five published systematic reviews (SR) focusing on the efficacy and safety of oral CHM for early stage DKD were identified. Two SRs only reported the meta-analysis results of effect rate, which was an unverified outcome.[1,2] Two other systematic reviews included studies with inappropriate controls, such as CM therapies as a comparator.[3,4] Therefore, only one published systematic review was consistent with the inclusion criteria and the results are highlighted here.[5]

In 2011, Xie *et al.* reported that oral CM formulae with tonifying *qi*, nourishing *yin* and activating Blood functions combined with angiotensin converting enzyme inhibitors (ACEi) or angiotensin receptor blockers (ARBs) was superior to ACEi/ARB alone in reducing albuminuria excretion rate (AER) and controlling blood glucose levels.[5] The meta-analysis included 16 randomised controlled trials (RCTs) with 1,159 participants with type 2 diabetes complicated by DKD with microalbuminuria. Three cases of adverse events (dry cough) were reported in one-study. However, unclear randomisation procedures and lack of blinding in the original studies may have introduced bias. In addition, meta-analysis of key outcomes showed high heterogeneity, the reasons for which were not identified. Therefore, the authors suggested that the results of these systematic reviews should be interpreted cautiously, such that rigorously designed and performed RCTs were conducted in the future to better understand the effects of CHM.

Identification of Clinical Studies

The study selection process is shown in Fig. 5.1. Comprehensive database searches identified more than 38,000 citations. After removing duplicates, screening irrelevant citations, and excluding citations according to exclusion criteria (see Chapter 4) a total of 464 clinical studies investigating the effects of CHM for DKD were included. Among all these clinical studies, 437 were RCTs (H1–H437), three were non-randomised controlled clinical trials (CCTs) (H438–H440), and 24 were non-controlled studies (H441–H464). RCTs and CCTs

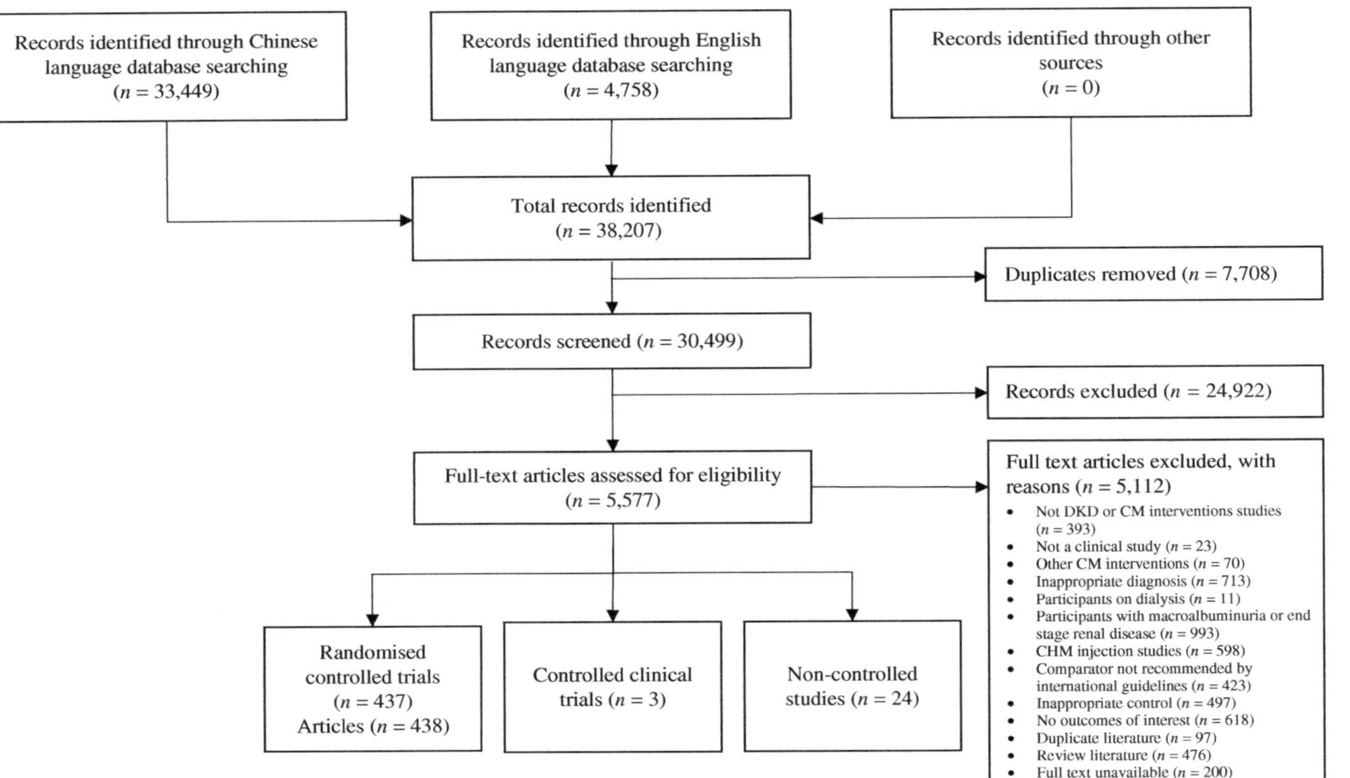

Fig. 5.1. Flow chart of study selection process: Chinese herbal medicine.

were grouped according to study design and comparison and included in the systematic review and meta-analysis. Information from non-controlled studies was summarised, including the characteristics of the study, details of the intervention and any adverse events. Non-controlled studies were not included in the quantitative analysis.

Oral Chinese Herbal Medicine

All 464 included studies applied CHM interventions in addition to conventional treatments (CTs), including various combinations of diet and lifestyle management, blood glucose control, blood pressure (BP) control and/or blood lipid control. In this monograph, CT included the antihypertensive agents other than ACEi or ARBs to control blood pressure (BP). Almost all CHM treatments were orally administered, except one study (H1) which treated participants with the combinations of oral and rectal CHM. Study results were analysed and presented in separate sections according to study design, that is, RCTs, CCTs, and non-controlled studies.

Randomised Controlled Trials of Oral Chinese Herbal Medicine

A total of 437 RCTs assessing CHM for DKD met the inclusion criteria (H1–H437). One study was conducted in Singapore (H2), and the others in China. The studies enrolled 31,301 patients with DKD and microalbuminuria (moderately increased albuminuria) aged between 18 and 89 years old (mean 55.6 years old). Except for 182 studies without information on primary cause, most of the studies ($n = 245$) enrolled participants with a primary cause of type 2 diabetes, and 10 studies enrolled participants with a primary cause of either type 1 or type 2 diabetes. Treatment durations of the studies widely ranged from two weeks to 24 months, with a median and mode of three months. Only six studies followed up the participants after completion of treatment. Three of them were followed up for six months (H3–H5), two for one year (H6, H7), and one for four weeks after the end of treatment (H8).

The majority of the studies had a two-arm parallel group design comparing oral CHM to CT or comparing oral CHM with a positive control of ACEi or ARBs. Twenty five (25) multiple-arm design studies compared oral CHM with CT as well as a positive control. Studies with multiple intervention groups were extracted and analysed in pairwise comparisons between all possible pairs of intervention groups. However, pairs which shared the same group were not included in the same meta-analysis.[6]

CM syndrome differentiation was used in 177 studies. One study allocated treatments according to individual syndrome differentiation (H9). The other 176 studies diagnosed specific syndromes as part of the study inclusion criteria. Symptoms reported in studies with non-standard symptom terms were standardised and grouped into categories. The specified syndromes, sorted from high to low frequencies, are presented in Table 5.1.

The 437 RCTs evaluated 338 different formulae and 235 different herbs. Among these formulae, 40 were unnamed and many were self-prescribed according to CM treatment principles. The formulae tested in multiple RCTs were traditional formulae (standard or modified) as well as commercial products. *Dong chong xia cao* preparation 冬虫夏草制剂 (a commercial product) was tested in 29 studies, which was the most frequently used CHM treatment. The most frequent formulae were *Liu wei di huang wan* 六味地黄丸 and

Table 5.1. Syndromes in Randomised Controlled Trials

Syndromes	No. of Studies
Qi and/or *yin* deficiency with Blood stasis	93
Spleen and/or Kidney deficiency with Blood stasis	33
Qi and/or *yin* deficiency	25
Spleen and/or Kidney deficiency	14
Liver and Kidney *yin* deficiency with Blood stasis	4
Yin and *yang* deficiency	3
Blood stasis	3
Liver and Kidney *yin* deficiency	1

Bu yang huan wu tang 补阳还五汤. Each was evaluated in eight studies (Table 5.2). In addition, many self-named and unnamed formulae were derived from, or had similar ingredients to, *Liu wei di huang wan* 六味地黄丸.

The largest formula comprised 21 herbs, but the average formula contained nine herbs. The commonly used herbs tested in more than 100 studies were *huang qi* 黄芪 (301 studies), *dan shen* 丹参 (209 studies), *shu di huang* 熟地黄 (203 studies), *shan yao* 山药 (152 studies), *shan zhu yu* 山茱萸 (145 studies), *fu ling* 茯苓 (118 studies), and *chuan xiong* 川芎 (107 studies) (Table 5.3). Almost half of the included studies used *huang qi* 黄芪, *dan shen* 丹参 and *shu di huang* 熟地黄.

Risk of Bias

All studies were described as "randomised", although only 86 studies (19.6%) reported an appropriate method for random sequence generation, and three studies (0.7%) described a non-random component in sequence generation i.e. odd or even visits. Only six studies (1.4%) reported that opaque envelopes were used to conceal allocation. Almost all the studies (98.2%) did not blind participants and investigators. None of the studies mention the blinding of outcome assessors. The majority of the studies (93.6%) did not have missing data or missing data were balanced in numbers with similar reasons across groups. Since the protocols of all included studies were not identified, insufficient information was available to judge whether the studies' reported outcomes were pre-specified. The overall methodological quality of the included RCTs was low (Table 5.4) and results should be interpreted with caution because of the risk of bias.

Outcomes

All four categories of the pre-defined primary outcomes including mortality, events indicating progression of disease, change in kidney function, and markers of kidney damage were reported, while several secondary outcomes, including cardiovascular mortality, all cause

Table 5.2. Frequently Used Oral Formulae in Randomised Controlled Trials

Most Common Formulae	No. of Studies	Standard Ingredients
Dong chong xia cao preparation 冬虫夏草制剂	29	*dong chong xia cao* (fermented *Cordyceps sinensis*) 发酵冬虫夏草菌丝
Liu wei di huang wan (including modified versions) 六味地黄丸(加减)	8	*fu ling* 茯苓, *shu di huang* 熟地黄, *shan yao* 山药, *shan zhu yu* 山茱萸, *mu dan pi* 牡丹皮, *ze xie* 泽泻
Bu yang huan wu tang (including modified versions) 补阳还五汤(加减)	8	*huang qi* 黄芪, *dang gui* 当归, *chi shao* 赤芍, *di long* 地龙, *chuang xiong* 川芎, *hong hua* 红花, *tao ren* 桃仁
Xue zhi kang capsule 血脂康胶囊	6	*hong qu* 红曲
Tong xin luo capsule 通心络胶囊	5	*ren shen* 人参, *shui zhi* 水蛭, *quan xie* 全蝎, *chi shao* 赤芍, *chan tui* 蝉蜕, *tu bie chong* 土鳖虫, *wu gong* 蜈蚣, *tan xiang* 檀香, *jiang xiang* 降香, *ru xiang* 乳香, *suan zao ren* 酸枣仁, *bing pian* 冰片
Shen qi di huang tang (including modified versions) 参芪地黄汤(加减)	4	*dang shen* 党参, *huang qi* 黄芪, *fu ling* 茯苓, *shu di huang* 熟地黄, *shan yao* 山药, *shan zhu yu* 山茱萸, *mu dan pi* 牡丹皮, *ze xie* 泽泻
Huang kui capsule 黄葵胶囊	4	*huang shu kui hua* 黄蜀葵花
Fu fang xue shuan tong capsule 复方血栓通胶囊	4	*san qi* 三七, *huang qi* 黄芪, *dan shen* 丹参, *xuan shen* 玄参
Niao du qing granule 尿毒清颗粒	4	*da huang* 大黄, *huang qi* 黄芪, *sang bai pi* 桑白皮, *ku shen* 苦参, *bai zhu* 白术, *fu ling* 茯苓, *bai shao* 白芍, *he shou wu* 何首乌, *dan shen* 丹参, *che qian cao* 车前草, etc.
Fu fang dan shen di wan 复方丹参滴丸	3	*dan shen* 丹参, *san qi* 三七, *bing pian* 冰片
Zhi tang bao shen granule 治糖保肾冲剂	3	*huang qi* 黄芪, *dan shen* 丹参, *da huang* 大黄, *shan zhu yu* 山茱萸, *ge gen* 葛根, *can jian* 蚕茧

(Continued)

Table 5.2.   (*Continued*)

Most Common Formulae	No. of Studies	Standard Ingredients
Yin xing ye preparations 银杏叶制剂	3	*yin xing ye* extraction 银杏叶提取物
Dan zhi jiang tang capsule 丹蛭降糖胶囊	2	*tai zi shen* 太子参, *di huang* 地黄, *mu dan pi* 牡丹皮, *ze xie* 泽泻, *shui zhi* 水蛭, *tu si zi* 菟丝子
Qi huang yin (modified) 加味芪黄饮	2	*tai zi shen* 太子参, *huang qi* 黄芪, *di huang* 地黄, *ze xie* 泽泻, *shan zhu yu* 山茱萸, *shan yao* 山药, *fu ling* 茯苓, *mu dan pi* 牡丹皮, *chan tui* 蝉蜕, *xi huang cao* 溪黄草, *nu zhen zi* 女贞子, *bai mao gen* 白茅根
Jin kui shen qi wan 金匮肾气丸	2	*gui zhi* 桂枝, *fu zi* 附子, *shan yao* 山药, *shan zhu yu* 山茱萸, *shu di huang* 熟地黄, *fu ling* 茯苓, *ze xie* 泽泻, *mu dan pi* 牡丹皮
Nao xin tong capsule 脑心通胶囊	2	*huang qi* 黄芪, *chi shao* 赤芍, *dan shen* 丹参, *dang gui* 当归, *chuan xiong* 川芎, *hong hua* 红花, *tao ren* 桃仁, *ru xiang* 乳香, *mo yao* 没药, *ji xue teng* 鸡血藤, *niu xi* 牛膝, *gui zhi* 桂枝, *sang zhi* 桑枝, *di long* 地龙, *quan xie* 全蝎, *shui zhi* 水蛭
Qi shen yi qi di wan 芪参益气滴丸	2	*huang qi* 黄芪, *dan shen* 丹参, *san qi* 三七, *jiang xiang* oil 降香油
Qi yao xiao ke capsule 芪药消渴胶囊	2	*xi yang shen* 西洋参, *huang qi* 黄芪, *shan yao* 山药, *di huang* 地黄, *shan zhu yu* 山茱萸, *gou qi zi* 枸杞子, *mai dong* 麦冬, *zhi mu* 知母, *tian hua fen* 天花粉, *wu wei zi* 五味子, *wu bei zi* 五倍子, *ge gen* 葛根
Shen yan kang fu pian 肾炎康复片	2	*xi yang shen* 西洋参, *ren shen* 人参, *di huang* 地黄, *du zhong* 杜仲, *shan yao* 山药, *bai hua she she cao* 白花蛇舌草, *tu fu ling* 土茯苓, *yi mu cao* 益母草, *dan shen* 丹参, *ze xie* 泽泻, *bai mao gen* 白茅根, *jie geng* 桔梗, *hei dou* 黑豆

Ingredients are referenced to the original studies where possible. If herb ingredients varied across studies, the herb ingredients were sourced from *Zhong Yi Fang Ji Da Ci Dian* 中医方剂大辞典.

Note: The use of some herbs may be restricted in some countries; readers are advised to comply with relevant regulations.

Table 5.3.   Frequently Reported Herbs in Randomised Controlled Trials

Most Common Herbs	Scientific Name	No. of Studies
Huang qi 黄芪	*Astragalus membranaceus* (Fisch.) Bge.	301
Dan shen 丹参	*Salvia miltiorrhiza* Bge.	209
(Shu) di huang (熟)地黄	*Rehmannia glutinosa* Libosch.	203
Shan yao 山药	*Dioscorea opposita* Thunb.	152
Shan zhu yu 山茱萸	*Cornus officinalis* Sieb. & Zucc.	145
Fu ling 茯苓	*Poria cocos* (Schw.) Wolf	118
Chuan xiong 川芎	*Ligusticum chuanxiong* Hort.	107
Da huang 大黄	*Rheum palmatum* L.; *Rheum tanguticum* Maxim. Ex Balf.; *Rheum officinale* Baill.	93
Dang gui 当归	*Angelica sinensis* (Oliv.) Diels	93
Ze xie 泽泻	*Alisma orientalis* (Sam.) Juzep.; *Alisma plantago-aquatica* L.	84
Shui zhi 水蛭	*Hirudo* or *Whitmania* spp.	68
Yi mu cao 益母草	*Leonurus japonicus* Houtt.	67
Bai zhu 白术	*Atractylodes macrocephala* Koidz.	65
Gou qi zi 枸杞子	*Lycium barbarum* L.	56
Ge gen 葛根	*Pueraria lobata* (Willd.) Ohwi	54
Qian shi 芡实	*Euryale ferox* Salisb.	54
Chi shao 赤芍	*Paeonia lactiflora* Pall.	51
Mu dan pi 牡丹皮	*Paeonia suffruticosa* Andr.	51
Tai zi shen 太子参	*Pseudostellaria heterophylla* (Miq.) Pax ex Pax et Hoffm.	51
Jin ying zi 金樱子	*Rosa laevigata* Michx.	49
Dang shen 党参	*Codonopsis pilosula* (Franch.) Nannf.	48
Hong hua 红花	*Carthamus tinctorius* L.	48

Note: The use of some herbs may be restricted in some countries; readers are advised to comply with relevant regulations.

hospitalisation and health care costs, were not reported in any studies. Nevertheless, because the study durations in most of these RCTs were not long enough to observe patient-level outcomes including mortality and events indicating disease progression, laboratory tests evaluating

Table 5.4. Risk of Bias of Randomised Controlled Trials

Risk of Bias Domain	Low Risk n (%)	Unclear Risk n (%)	High Risk n (%)
Sequence generation	86 (19.6%)	348 (76.7%)	3 (0.7%)
Allocation concealment	6 (1.4%)	428 (98.0%)	3 (0.7%)
Blinding of participants	8 (1.8%)	0 (0%)	429 (98.2%)
Blinding of personnel	3 (0.7%)	5 (1.1%)	429 (98.2%)
Blinding of outcome assessors	0 (0%)	437 (100%)	0 (0%)
Incomplete outcome data	409 (93.6%)	27 (6.2%)	1 (0.2%)
Selective outcome reporting	0 (0%)	423 (96.8%)	14 (3.2%)

blood and urine markers of kidney damage were the most commonly reported outcomes.

In the following sections, the analysis results are presented by outcome measures. Each outcome is grouped according to the type of comparison as follows:

- CHM plus CT vs. CT (plus CHM placebo)
- CHM plus CT vs. CT plus ACEi or ARBs
- CHM plus CT plus ACEi or ARBs vs. CT plus ACEi or ARBs (plus CHM placebo)

All included studies assessed CHM interventions added to CTs including various combinations of diet and lifestyle managements, blood glucose control, BP control and/or blood lipid control.

Subgroup analysis was conducted according to additional factors, including CM formulae, treatment duration, and baseline kidney function.

All-cause Mortality and Disease Progression

CHM Plus Benazepril Plus CT vs. Benazepril Plus CT

In a study including 70 participants and comparing oral CHM plus benazepril with benazepril for three months, no fatal events were observed during the study period, while kidney survival analysis showed that disease progression (defined as commencement of dialysis) improved in the CHM group (92.1% vs. 75.0%, Log-rank test, $X^2 = 4.23$, $P = 0.04$) (H10).

CHM Plus CT vs. Irbesartan Plus CT

In another study that included 78 participants and compared oral CHM with irbesartan for one year, no significant difference was observed between groups with respect to the event of albuminuria progression (from micro- to macro-albuminuria) (RR 0.51 [0.1, 2.64]) (H11).

Other events indicating progression, such as progressing to end-stage renal disease (ESRD), doubling of serum creatinine (SCr) from baseline, percentage decline in glomerular filtration rate (GFR) or estimated GFR (eGFR) and change in chronic kidney disease (CKD) stage, were not reported in included studies.

Glomerular Filtration Rate (GFR) and Estimated GFR

CHM Plus CT vs. CT

Compared to CTs, one study including 50 participants reported that oral CHM as an integrative treatment for three months improved GFR (measured by single-photon emission computed tomography) (mean difference (MD) 15.8mL/min [6.5, 25.12]) (H12). However, pooled results from another eight RCTs (8 weeks to six months) showed no significant difference in eGFR-Cockcroft-Gault (patients with supranormal GFR (mean eGFR estimated by the Cockcroft-Gault equation over 130mL/min) between groups (MD −6.99mL/min [−15.41, 1.43], $I^2 = 92.8\%$) (H13–H20).

CHM Plus ACEi/ARBs Plus CT vs. ACEi/ARBs Plus CT

In 19 RCTs that compared CHM plus an ACEi or ARBs with an ACEi or ARBs (4 weeks to 12 months), there was no significant difference in eGFR-Cockcroft-Gault (MD −4.07mL/min [−10.28, 2.14], $I^2 = 97.6\%$)

at the end of treatment (H5, H21–H38). A trend of improvement was found in the subgroup of more than three months treatment, although this result was not significantly different: less than three months treatment (MD –7.03mL/min [–14.96, 0.90], I^2 = 98%), more than three months treatment (MD 3.33mL/min [–4.22, 10.88], I^2 = 89%). The results were consistent with the sensitivity analysis of RCTs judged as low risk on the basis for sequence generation (MD –3.25mL/min [–20.38, 13.89], I^2 = 96.2%) (H31, H33, H37).

CHM Plus CT vs. ACEi/ARBs Plus CT

Three studies assessed the effects of CHM for early DKD patients with supranormal GFR. For two RCTs that compared CHM with losartan for two to three months, eGFR decreased to the normal range at the end of treatment in both groups, although there was no significant difference between the groups (MD –1.35mL/min [–17.16, 14.45], I^2 = 93%) (H39, H40). Results from one double dummy placebo-controlled study involving 90 participants showed that oral CHM produced an additional reduction of eGFR compared to benazepril (MD –1.14mL/min [–1.58, –0.69]) (H41).

Serum Creatinine

CHM Plus CT vs. CT

Pooled results from 32 RCTs showed that CHM plus CT reduced SCr (MD –8.57μmol/L [–13.30, –3.85], I^2 = 96.2%) (H13, H16, H17, H19, H42–H69). In the subgroups of treatment durations, results showed that longer treatment (≥ three months) produced a larger effect. Amongst the subgroups of different baseline kidney function, a significant difference was only found in the subgroup of GFR ≥ 60 mL/min, but not in the subgroup of GFR < 60mL/min. (Table 5.5).

CHM Plus ACEi/ARBs Plus CT vs. ACEi/ARBs Plus CT

Over 100 RCTs enrolled 7,501 participants and evaluated the combinations of oral CHM and an ACEi or oral CHM and an ARB. The

Table 5.5. Oral Chinese Herbal Medicine Plus Conventional Treatment vs. Conventional Treatment: SCr (μmol/L)

Total/Subgroups	No. of Studies (Duration)	No. of Participants	MD [95% CI]	I^2%	Included Studies
Total	32 (2w–6m)	2,319	−8.57 [−13.30, −3.85]*	96.2%	H13, H16, H17, H19, H42–H69
Subgroup: Td < 3m	16 (2w–8w)	1,119	−2.95 [−5.63, −0.27]*	67.0%	H13, H16, H17, H19, H42–H45, H47, H49, H51, H54, H55, H57, H59, H69
Sub: Td ≥ 3m	19 (3m–6m)	1,200	−13.72 [−20.55, −6.90]*	96.5%	H46, H48, H50, H52, H53, H56, H58, H60–H68
Sub: Baseline GFR ≥ 60mL/min	8 (2w–3m)	537	−5.95 [−10.74, −1.16]*	89.7%	H42, H43, H54, H57, H63, H68, H70, H71
Sub: Baseline GFR < 60mL/min	2 (8w–6m)	144	−25.47 [−77.61, 26.66]	99.5%	H19, H46

*Statistically significant.

Abbreviatons: CHM, Chinese herbal medicine; CT, conventional treatments; MD, mean difference; SCr, serum creatinine; GFR, glomerular filtration rate.

overall meta-analysis showed that oral CHM plus ACEi or ARBs was superior to ACEi or ARBs alone in terms of SCr reduction (MD −5.95μmol/L [−8.09, −3.82], I^2 = 92.9%). The pooled results of the combination of CHM and ACEi and the combination of ARBs were consistent with the overall pooled result (Table 5.6). The additional effect on SCr reduction was found in the subgroup of baseline GFR less than 60mL/min but not in the subgroup of more than 60mL/min (Table 5.6). It suggests that the combination of CHM and ACEi or ARB was beneficial for DKD patients at advanced stages (CKD G3–G5), while the effect in early stage of CKD was unclear.

CHM Plus CT vs. ACEi/ARBs Plus CT

Twenty-one (21) RCTs used conventional treatments plus ACEi or ARBs as comparators for six to 24 weeks with 1,580 participants enrolled. At the end of treatment, there was no significant difference between the CHM and ACEi or ARB groups in SCr reduction (MD −0.10 μmol/L [−2.06, 1.86], I^2 = 53%). Two different trends were shown in the results of subgroup analysis. A slight decrease in SCr was observed in a subgroup with treatment durations of more than three months and in a subgroup with baseline GFR more than 60mL/min, while an opposite trend was observed in a subgroup with treatment durations less than three months and a subgroup with baseline GFR less than 60mL/min (Table 5.7). Although there were no significant differences in any of the subgroups, the results raise the possibility that CHM has a greater effect on SCr reduction with longer treatment duration and in DKD patients at early stages (i.e. CKD G1 and G2).

Albuminuria and Proteinuria

CHM Plus CT vs. (CHM Placebo Plus) CT

The mean differences in AER before and after CT alone were −21.29mg/24h, and −18.92μg/min. Pooled results from RCTs which did not use placebo showed that CHM appeared to have additional

Table 5.6. Oral Chinese Herbal Medicine Plus ACEi/ARBs Plus Conventional Treatment vs. ACEi/ARBs Plus Conventional Treatment: SCr (μmol/L)

Total/ Subgroups	No. of Studies (Duration)	No. of Participants	MD [95% CI]	I^2%	Included Studies
Total	105 (2w–6m)	7,501	−5.95 [−8.09, −3.82]*	92.9%	H4, H9, H11, H21, H23–H25, H27, H29–H31, H33–H35, H63, H69, H72–H160
Subgroup: combined with ACEi	45 (2w–6m)	3,160	−7.68 [−11.82, −3.53]*	94.9%	H4, H21, H23, H25, H27, H30, H31, H33, H35, H73, H76, H77, H79, H81, H82, H84, H86–H88, H90, H92, H98, H104, H106, H113, H115, H117, H118, H121, H127, H128, H132, H136–H139, H142, H143, H146–H148, H153, H158–H160
Sub: combined with ARBs	51 (2w–6m)	3,675	−5.14 [−7.77, −2.51]*	91.3%	H9, H11, H24, H29, H34, H63, H69, H72, H75, H80, H83, H85, H89, H91, H93–H96, H97, H100, H101, H103, H105, H107–H112, H114, H119, H120, H122–H125, H130, H131, H133–H135, H140, H141, H144, H145, H149–H151, H154–H156
Sub: Td < 3m	50 (2w–8w)	3,621	−5.53 [−9.15, −1.92]*	95.3%	H9, H23, H25, H29, H33, H35, H69, H72, H74, H77, H82, H84, H86, H89, H92, H98, H99, H104, H106, H109, H110, H113, H116, H120, H121, H123, H125, H128, H129, H135, H139, H141, H143, H144, H146, H148–H150, H153, H157, H159

(*Continued*)

Table 5.6. (*Continued*)

Total/ Subgroups	No. of Studies (Duration)	No. of Participants	MD [95% CI]	I²%	Included Studies
Sub: Td ≥ 3m	53 (3w–6m)	3,797	−6.54 [−8.98, −4.09]*	87.2%	H4, H21, H27, H30, H31, H34, H63, H73, H75, H76, H78–H81, H83, H85, H87, H88, H93–H96, H97, H100–H103, H107, H108, H111, H112, H114, H115, H117–H119, H122, H127, H130–H134, H140, H142, H145, H147, H151, H152, H154–H156, H158
Sub: Baseline GFR ≥ 60mL/min	18 (6w–6m)	1,330	0.06 [−2.37, 2.48]	57.6%	H23, H23, H63, H72, H81, H88, H93, H94, H98, H108–H110, H124, H128, H133, H140, H141, H156, H158
Sub: Baseline GFR < 60mL/min	7 (12w–6m)	482	−6.98 [−12.48, −1.48]*	82.9%	H85, H89, H103, H119, H131, H132, H152

*Statistically significant.

Abbreviations: ACEi, angiotensin converting enzyme inhibitors; ARBs, angiotensin II receptor blockers; GFR, glomerular filtraction rate; MD, mean difference; Td, treatment duration.

Table 5.7. Oral Chinese Herbal Medicine Plus Conventional Treatment vs. ACEi/ARBs Plus Conventional Treatment: SCr (μmol/L)

Total/Subgroups	No. of Studies (Duration)	No. of Participants	MD [95% CI]	I^2%	Included Studies
Total	21 (6w–24w)	1,580	−0.10 [−2.06, 1.86]	53%	H39, H40, H46, H63, H69, H73, H128, H140, H143, H147, H161–H163, H164, H165, H166, H167, H168–H171
Subgroup: Td < 3m	9 (6w–2m)	630	1.38 [−2.08, 4.85]	62%	H39, H69, H128, H143, H161, H162, H164, H168, H169
Sub: Td ≥ 3m	12 (3–6m)	950	−1.13 [−3.33, 1.07]	39%	H40, H46, H63, H73, H140, H147, H163, H165–H167, H170, H171
Sub: Baseline GFR ≥ 60mL/min	5 (8w–3m)	332	−0.02 [−1.99, 1.95]	0%	H63, H128, H140, H164, H166
Sub: Baseline GFR < 60mL/min	2 (12–24w)	251	0.78 [−2.79, 4.34]	0%	H46, H163

Abbreviations: MD, mean difference; SCr, serum creatinine; Td, treatment duration; GFR, glomerular filtration rate.

benefit on albuminuria and proteinuria reduction in terms of AER, albumin to creatinine ratio (ACR), urinary albuminuria concentration (UAC) and urinary protein excretion (UPE) (Table 5.8). However, the data demonstrated considerable statistical heterogeneity.

Moreover, when compared to placebo, the additional effect of CHM on albuminuria and proteinuria reduction was uncertain. In two 12-week RCTs, CHM reduced AER (MD −52.17mg/24h [−68.34, −35.99], I^2 = 50.7%) (H172, H173). On the other hand, in two randomised double-blind placebo-controlled trials of one to two years duration, a significant add-on benefit of CHM in terms of ACR reduction was not found (MD −30.53mg/g [−76.59, 15.53], I^2 = 66%) (H174, H175).

One placebo-controlled study reported that there was no difference on UPE between groups at the end of three months treatment (MD −18.0mg/L [−53.92, 17.92]) (H176).

CHM Plus ACEi/ARBs Plus CT vs. ACEi/ARBs Plus CT

Two hundred and forty seven (247) RCTs investigated the renal protective effects of the combinations of CHM and ACEi as well as CHM and ARBs. The mean differences in AER before and after ACEi/ARBs plus CT were −45mg/24h, and −34.11µg/min. Pooled results showed that combination treatment produced further reductions in albuminuria and proteinuria compared to ACEi or ARBs (Table 5.9). The results were consistent among various laboratory methods of albuminuria, i.e. measurement of UAC, measurement of ACR and AER on spot urine and AER on timed urine collection (24 hours is the most common timed collection period used in China).

CHM Plus CT vs. ACEi/ARBs Plus CT

Pooled results from 66 RCTs showed that, when added to CTs, CHM was superior to ACEi or ARBs with respect to albuminuria and proteinuria reduction (Table 5.10). Sensitivity analysis of RCTs which were at low risk of bias in terms of sequence generation demonstrated consistent results for AER. It should be noted that blinding was

Table 5.8. **Oral Chinese Herbal Medicine Plus Conventional Treatment vs. Conventional Treatment (with or without placebo): Albuminuria and Proteinuria**

Intervention	Comparator	Outcome (Unit)	No. of Studies (Duration)	No. of Participants	MD [95% CI]	I²	Included Studies
Oral CHM + CTs	CTs	ACR (mg/g)	3 (3w–6m)	212	−51.14 [−81.24, −21.04]*	97.3%	H64, H68, H402
		AER (mg/24h)	32 (1m–6m)	2,003	−49.97 [−59.31,−40.63]*	96.7%	H2, H13, H14, H17, H19, H53, H54, H59, H60, H63, H67, H70, H71, H177–H195
		AER (µg/min)	49 (2w–6m)	3,280	−40.66 [−53.86,−27.47]*	99.4%	H15, H18, H20, H42–H47, H49, H51, H52, H55, H56, H58, H61, H62, H66, H196–H226
		UAC (mg/L)	7 (2w–3m)	560	−26.13 [−33.98, −18.29]*	99.7%	H44, H48, H51, H68, H199, H226–H234
		UPE (mg/24h)	14 (1–4m)	907	−83.32 [−117.58, −49.06]*	99.1%	H44, H48, H51, H68, H199, H226–H234
	Placebo + CTs	ACR (mg/g)	2 (1–2y)	124	−30.53 [−76.59, 15.53]	66%	H174, H175
		AER (mg/24h)	2 (12w)	198	−52.17 [−68.34, −35.99]*	50.7%	H172, H173
		UPE (mg/L)	1 (3m)	23	−18.0 [−53.92, 17.92]	NA.	H176

*Statistically significant.

Abbreviations: ACR, albumin to creatinine ratio; AER, albumin excretion rate; CHM, Chinese herbal medicine; CT, conventional treatments; MD, mean difference; UAC, urinary albuminuria concentration; UPE, urinary protein excretion; NA, not applicable.

Table 5.9. Oral Chinese Herbal Medicine Plus ACEi/ARBs Plus Conventional Treatment vs. ACEi/ARBs Plus Conventional Treatment: Albuminuria and Proteinuria

Outcome (unit)	No. of Studies (duration)	No. of Participants	MD [95% CI]	I^2	Included Studies
ACR (mg/g)	16 (4–24w)	1,142	−15.43 [−18.94, −11.93]*	71.1%	H23, H31, H37, H72, H87, H98, H141, H146, H235–H242
AER (mg/24h)	83 (2w–12m)	5,666	−34.29 [−38.62, −29.97]*	95.2%	H5, H22, H24, H25, H27, H28, H32, H33, H36, H38, H63, H74, H80, H85–H89, H96, H99, H103, H106, H110, H113, H114, H116, H118, H120, H122, H126, H130, H131, H133, H144, H145, H147, H148, H152, H156, H187, H235, H238, H243–H283
AER (µg/min)	102 (2w–6m)	7,601	−24.79 [−27.24, −22.36]*	94.9%	H4, H9, H11, H21, H29, H34, H35, H73, H76–H79, H82, H84, H90, H92–H95, H97, H100, H104, H105, H107–H109, H111, H115, H119, H121, H123, H124, H129, H135–H138, H140, H143, H149–H151, H153, H154, H155, H158, H242, H284–H338
UAC (mg/L)	16 (4–16w)	1,063	−25.64 [−32.57, −18.71]*	99.7%	H75, H91, H101, H102, H117, H125, H139, H157, H159, H339–H345
UPE (mg/24h)	44 (4w–6m)	3,167	−47.34 [−55.11, −39.58]*	96%	H7, H21, H24, H26, H29, H34, H37, H79, H81, H83, H87, H102, H110, H112, H125, H127, H132, H134, H136, H142, H149, H241, H242, H294, H298, H305, H311, H312, H316, H336–H338, H341, H344, H346–H355

*Statistically significant.

Abbreviations: ACEi, angiotensin converting enzyme inhibitor;; ACR, albumin to creatinine ratio; AER, albumin excretion rate; ARBs, angiotensin receptor blockers; MD, mean difference; UAC, urinary albuminuria concentration; UPE, urinary protein excretion.

Table 5.10. Oral Chinese Herbal Medicine Plus Conventional Treatment vs. ACEi/ARBs Plus Conventional Treatment: Albuminuria and Proteinuria

Intervention	Comparator	Outcome (unit)	No. of Studies	No. of Participants	MD [95% CI]	I^2	Included Studies
Oral CHM + benazepril placebo	Benazepril + CHM placebo	AER (mg/24h)	1 (2m)	90	−44.55 [−47.03, −42.07]*	NA	H41
Oral CHM	ACEi or ARBs	ACR (mg/g)	3 (8w–3m)	196	−28.84 [−36.89, −20.78]*	0%	H379, H418, H437
		AER (mg/24h)	32 (4w–12m)	2,117	−24.79 [−30.99, −18.59]*	92%	H3, H63, H70, H71, H147, H161, H164, H170, H180, H183, H187, H247, H253, H356, H357, H358–H360, H361, H362, H363–H365, H366, H367, H368, H369–H374
		AER (µg/min)	35 (4–16w)	2,470	−18.25 [−23.25, −13.26]*	96%	H39, H40, H46, H73, H140, H143, H165, H166, H168, H171, H223, H224, H288, H309, H332, H375, H376, H377–H394
		UAC (mg/L)	2 (12w)	271	−26.00 [−57.41, 5.41]	99%	H163, H379
		UPE (mg/24h)	6 (8–12w)	446	−46.68 [−78.49, −14.86]*	95%	H39, H161, H169, H377, H395, H396

*Statistically significant.

Abbreviations: ACEi, angiotensin converting enzyme inhibitor, AER, albumin excretion rate; ARBs, angiotensin receptor blockers; CHM, Chinese herbal medicine; MD, mean difference; UAC, urinary albuminuria concentration, UPE, urinary protein excretion; NA, not applicable.

not performed in all studies included in the pooled estimation, and significant heterogeneity existed.

A double dummy placebo-controlled study that enrolled 90 patients with type 2 diabetes and persistent microalbuminuria aged 35–70 years old, compared CHM to benazepril. AER was significantly decreased in both the CHM and benazepril groups after a two-month treatment period, and a significant difference was found between the two groups (MD –44.55mg/24h [–47.03, –42.07]) (H41).

Blood Pressure

CHM Plus CT vs. (CHM Placebo Plus) CT

Several studies assessed BP after adding oral CHM to CTs (ACEi or ARBs not used for BP control). Five RCTs enrolled participants with baseline mean systolic BPs (SBPs) of 154 mmHg and 151mmHg and baseline mean diastolic BPs (DBPs) of 88 mmHg and 89 mmHg in the treatment and control groups, respectively. Mean SBP at the end of treatment in both groups did not reach the target of 140mmHg, and pooled results showed that there was no significant difference between groups in terms of lowering blood pressure (MD –1.95mmHg [–3.96, 0.06], $I^2 = 0$) (H44, H47, H69, H223, H224).

Two placebo-controlled RCTs enrolled participants whose BP reached the target values. Pooled results showed that BP remained within the target ranges at the end of treatment in both groups, and there was no significant difference between groups in terms of SBP (MD –1.10 mmHg [–5.48, 3.28], $I^2 = 0$) and DBP (MD 0.02 mmHg [–3.72, 3.76], $I^2 = 36\%$) (H174, H175).

CHM Plus ACEi/ARBs vs. ACEi/ARBs

Thirty seven (37) RCTs compared oral CHM plus ACEi or ARBs with ACEi or ARBs alone and reported BP measurements. The results were not consistent with respect to BP control. At the end of the combined treatment, SBP was reduced (MD –2.06 mmHg [–3.09, –1.03], $I^2 = 69.9\%$) while there was no significant difference in DBP (MD –0.81mmHg

[–1.90, 0.29], I^2 = 84.3%) or mean artery pressure (MD 0.88 mmHg [–1.14, 2.89], I^2 = 33.8%) (H72, H76, H98, H398).

CHM vs. ACEi/ARBs

Eight (8) RCTs that compared oral CHM with ACEi or ARBs measured BP in 504 participants. Both SBP and DBP significantly decreased with the treatments of CHM and ACEi/ARBs (CHM: SBP: MD –5.98 [–10.03, –1.92], I^2 = 70%; DBP: MD –3.25 [–4.70, –1.80], I^2 = 23%; ACEi/ARBs: SBP: MD –10.07 [–17.61, –2.52], I^2 = 90%; DBP: MD –4.05 [–7.85, –0.25], I^2 = 76%). However, ACEi or ARBs were superior to CHM with respect to BP lowering (SBP: MD 4.28 mmHg [0.52, 8.04], I^2 = 66%; DBP: MD 1.12 mmHg [–0.92, 3.16], I^2 = 30%).

Blood Glucose and Blood Lipids

In order to evaluate the effects of oral CHM in terms of blood glucose lowering and lipid regulation, all included RCTs which reported outcomes for glucose and lipid levels were regrouped and pooled into a meta-analysis as follows:

Blood Glucose

- CHM plus hypoglycaemic agents *vs.* hypoglycaemic agents (plus CHM placebo)

Blood lipids

- CHM *vs.* placebo
- CHM *vs.* no lipid-lowering agents
- CHM plus lipid-lowering agents *vs.* lipid-lowering agents

Blood Glucose

CHM Plus Hypoglycaemic Agents vs. CHM Placebo Plus Hypoglycaemic Agents

Four RCTs compared oral CHM with placebo as an adjunct to hypoglycaemic agents for eight weeks to 24 months. The mean baseline fasting blood glucose (FBG) levels were 7.58mmol/L in the combination group and 7.61mmol/L in the hypoglycaemic agents group. At the end of treatment, there was no significant difference between the two groups with respect to both FBG (MD −0.84mmol/L [−2.39, 0.71], I^2 = 96.7%) (H173–H175, H399) and haemoglobin A1c (HbA1c) (MD 0.15% [−0.30, 0.60]) (H175).

CHM Plus Hypoglycaemic Agents vs. Hypoglycaemic Agents

Two hundred and thirty four (234) RCTs evaluated the effect of adding oral CHM to hypoglycaemic agents compared to hypoglycaemic agents alone. These studies enrolled 16,001 participants with a mean baseline FBG of 8.9mmol/L and a mean baseline HbA1c of 8.4%. FBG and HbA1c decreased in both groups at the end of treatment compared to baseline levels. The overall pooled result showed that oral CHM as an integrative treatment may produce a superior hypoglycaemic effect, as determined by FBG (MD −0.44mmol/L [−0.51, −0.36], I^2 = 88.4%) and HbA1c (MD −0.44% [−0.5,−0.35], I^2 = 95.8%).

In the subgroup-analyses according to mean baseline FBG (≥ 6 and < 6mmol/L) and HbA1c (≥ 6.5% and < 6.5%), FBG and HbA1c% both decreased within groups. A more profound hypoglycaemic effect was observed in the subgroups of mean baseline FBG ≥ 6mmol/L and HbA1c ≥ 6.5% between groups, but not in the subgroups of mean baseline FBG < 6mmol/L and HbA1c < 6.5%. These results suggest that oral CHM plus hypoglycaemic agents may be superior, or at least not inferior, to hypoglycaemic agents alone in lowering blood glucose.

Blood Lipids

CHM vs. Placebo

Pooled results from four placebo-controlled RCTs showed that oral CHM treatment for 8–12 weeks reduced blood lipids in terms of total cholesterol (TC) (MD −1.32mmol/L [−2.40, −0.25], I^2 = 97.1%), low-density lipoprotein (LDL) cholesterol (MD −0.77mmol/L [−1.50, −0.04], I^2 = 96.7%) and triglycerides (TG) (MD −0.99mmol/L [−1.61, −0.37], I^2 = 95.3%) compared to placebo (H172, H173, H175, H399).

CHM vs. no Lipid-lowering Agents

A total of 126 RCTs compared oral CHM with no lipid-lowering agents. Pooled results showed that total cholesterol (TC) (MD −0.81mmol/L [−0.94, −0.68], I^2 = 97%), TG (MD −0.61mmol/L [−0.69, −0.52], I^2 = 96.1%) and LDL (MD −0.54mmol/L [−0.70, −0.38], I^2 = 92.7%) were reduced, and high-density lipoprotein (HDL) (MD 0.22mmol/L [0.16, 0.27], I^2 = 95.4%) was increased with oral CHM treatment.

CHM Plus Lipid-lowering Agents vs. Lipid-lowering Agents

Pooled results from 33 RCTs showed that adding oral CHM to lipid-lowering agents may produce an additional blood lipid lowering effect. At the end of integrative treatment, TC (MD −0.58mmol/L [−0.87, −0.29], I^2 = 95.9%), TG (MD −0.5.3mmol/L [−0.77, −0.28], I^2 = 96.9%) and LDL (MD −0.45mmol/L [−0.61, −0.29], I^2 = 89.7%) were reduced, and HDL was increased (MD 0.20mmol/L [0.07, 0.32], I^2 = 91.7%).

Quality of Life

Two studies evaluated the quality of life of the enrolled participants. One study mentioned that they used a diabetes-specific quality of life scale in the methods section but did not report any results (H135). The other study that compared oral CHM plus valsartan with valsartan alone suggested that total scores of quality of life were significantly improved in both groups after treatments, and the improvement in the combination group was superior to that of the valsartan group (H141). However, it was difficult to assess the effect as the study did not report the scale that was used to evaluate quality of life.

Assessment Using Grading of Recommendations Assessment, Development and Evaluation (GRADE)

An assessment of the quality of the evidence from RCTs was made using Grading of Recommendations Assessment, Development and Evaluation (GRADE). Interventions, comparators and outcomes were selected based on a consensus process, described in Chapter 4. Comparisons were:

1. CHM plus CTs versus (placebo plus) CTs (Table 5.11);
2. CHM plus CTs versus ACEi/ARB plus CTs (Table 5.12);
3. CHM plus CTs and ACEi/ARB versus CTs and ACEi/ARB (Table 5.13);
4. CHM plus CTs versus ACEi/ARB plus CTs (Table 5.14); and
5. CHM plus CTs plus ACEi placebo versus placebo CHM plus CTs plus ACEi (Table 5.15).

1. *CHM Plus CT vs. CT*

Evidence for CHM plus CTs compared to CTs was very low to low quality (Table 5.11). The results showed that oral CHM plus CTs may reduce SCr and albuminuria and may slightly improve eGFR (low certainty evidence).

2. *CHM Plus CT vs. Placebo CHM Plus CT*

Evidence from trials evaluating CHM plus CT compared to placebo CHM plus CT were low quality (Table 5.12). The effect on reducing albuminuria excretion was uncertain, and further high quality studies are needed. Other primary outcomes were not reported.

3. *CHM Plus CT Plus ACEi/ARBs vs. ACEi/ARBs Plus CT*

Evidence from studies of CHM plus ACEi or ARBs plus CTs were of very low to low quality (Table 5.13). The effect of combination

Table 5.11.   GRADE: Oral Chinese Herbal Medcine Plus Conventional Treatment vs. Conventional Treatment

Outcomes	GRADE	Risk with CTs	Anticipated Absolute Effects
			Risk Difference with CHM and CTs
All-cause mortality, progression to ESRD, and change in CKD stage			Not measured
eGFR-Cockcroft-Gault Td: mean 9 weeks N = 588 (8 RCTs)	⊕◯◯◯ VERY LOW[1,2,3]	The mean eGFR was 99.03 mL/min	MD 6.99 mL/min lower (15.41 lower to 1.43 higher)
SCr Td: mean 11.25 weeks N = 2.319 (32 RCTS)	⊕⊕◯◯ LOW[1,2]	The mean SCr was 98.02 µmol/L	MD 8.57 µmol/L lower (13.3 lower to 3.85 lower)
Albuminuria Assessed with: ACR Td: mean 13.33 weeks N = 212 (3 RCTs)	⊕◯◯◯ VERY LOW[1,2,4]	The mean ACR was 136.3 mg/g	MD 51.14 mg/g lower (81.24 lower to 21.04 lower)
Adverse events N = 2,488 (37 RCTs)	A total of 29 studies reported that no adverse events occurred. Eight studies reported a small number of events such as abdominal discomfort, nausea, vomiting, loose stools/diarrhoea, or dark/black stools after CHM. Hypoglycaemia was reported in the control group.		

The risk in the intervention group (and its 95% CI) is based on the assumed risk in the comparison group and the relative effect of the intervention (and its 95% CI). 1. Unclear sequence generation and allocation concealment. Lack of blinding of participants and personnel. 2. Considerable statistical heterogeneity. 3. Wide confidence interval. 4. Small sample size.

Abbreviations: ACR, albumin to creatinine ratio; CHM, Chinese herbal medicine; CI, confidence interval; CKD. chronic kidney disease; CT, conventional treatments; eGFR, estimated glomerular filtration rate; ESRD, end-stage renal disease: MD. mean difference: RCTs, randomised controlled trials; SCr, serum creatinine; Td: treatment duration.

Study References: eGFR: H13–H20; SCr: H13, H16, H17, HI9, H42–H69; SCr: H13, H16, H17. H19.H42- H69: Albuminuria: H64, H68, H402; Adverse events: HI9, H20, H43, H47, H53, H54, H56, H59, H64, H70, H71, H178, H181–H183, H185, H190, H191, H200, H201, H204, H205, H211, H212, H215, H218, H220, H221, H230, H232, H234, H407, H413, H415, H429, H430, H435.

Table 5.12   GRADE: Oral Chinese Herbal Medicine Plus Conventional Treatment vs. Placebo Chinese Herbal Medicine Plus Conventional Treatment

| | | Anticipated Absolute Effects | |
| | | Risk with Placebo | Risk Difference |
Outcomes	GRADE	CHM and CTs	with CHM and CTs
All-cause mortality, progression to ESRD, and change in CKD stage			Not measured
Albuminuria Assessed with: ACR Treatment duration: mean 13.33 weeks N = 124 (2 RCTs)	⊕⊕◯◯ LOW[1,2,3]	The mean ACR was 49.36 mg/g	MD 30.53 mg/g lower (76.59 lower to 15.53 higher)
Adverse events		Not reported	

The risk in the intervention group (and its 95% CI) is based on the assumed risk in the comparison group and the relative; effect of the intervention (and its 95% CI). 1. Unclear sequence generation and allocation concealment. 2. Considerable statistical heterogeneity. 3. Small sample size.

Abbreviations: ACR, albumin to creatinine ratio; CHM, Chinese herbal medicine; CI, Confidence interval; CT, conventional treatments;

MD: mean difference; RCTs: randomised controlled trials.

Study References: H174, H175

treatment on reducing the number of eventS of progressing to ESRD and number of events of albuminuria progression was uncertain, as was the effect on eGFR. However, the combined use of CHM with ACEi/ARB may lower the SCr concentration and albuminuria excretion more than ACEi/ARB alone (low certainty evidence).

4. *CHM Plus CT vs. ACEi/ARBs Plus CT*

Evidence for oral CHM plus CTs compared to ACEi or ARBs was very low to low quality (Table 5.14). The results showed that, compared to ACEi or ARBs, CHM plus CTs may reduce albuminuria (low certainty evidence). However, the effect of CHM versus ACEi or ARB on improving eGFR and SCr level was uncertain.

Table 5.13. GRADE: Chinese Herbal Medicine Plus Conventional Treatment Plus ACEi/ARB vs. Conventional Treatment Plus ACEi/ARB

Outcomes	GRADE	Anticipated Absolute Effects	
		Risk with CTs and ACEi/ARB	Risk Difference with CHM and CTs and ACEi/ARB
All-cause mortality Td: 90 days N = 70 (1 RCTs)	⊕⊕○○ LOW[1,2]	Not estimable — no events	
Progression to ESRD Td: 90 days N = 70 (1 RCTs)	⊕⊕○○ LOW[1,2]	211 per 1,000 (RR 0.45 (0.13 to 1.54))	116 fewer per 1,000 (183 fewer to 114 more)
Albuminuria progression Assessed with: from micro- to macro- Td: Not stated N = 75 (1 RCTs)	⊕⊕○○ LOW[1,2]	105 per 1,000 (RR 0.51 (0.10 to 2.64))	54 fewer per 1,000 (95 fewer to 173 more)
eGFR-Cockcroft-Gault Td: mean 11.58 weeks N = 1,191 (19 RCTs)	⊕○○○ VERY LOW[1,3,4]	The mean eGFR was 103.46 mL/min	MD 4.07 mL/min lower (10.28 lower to 2.14 higher)
SCr Td: mean 10.80 weeks N = 7,501 (105 RCTs)	⊕⊕○○ LOW[1,4]	The mean SCr was 92.18 μmol/L	MD 5.95 μmol/L lower (8.09 lower to 3.82 lower)
Albuminuria Assessed with: ACR Td: mean 10.13 weeks N = 1,142(16 RCTs)	⊕⊕○○ LOW[1,4]	The mean ACR was 95.78 mg/g	MD 15.43 mg/g lower (18.94 lower to 11.93 lower)

(Continued)

Table 5.13. (*Continued*)

Outcomes	GRADE	Anticipated Absolute Effects	
		Risk with CTs and ACEi/ARB	Risk Difference with CHM and CTs and ACEi/ARB
Adverse events N = 7,265 (100 RCTs)		A total of 76 studies reported that no adverse events occurred. A total of 24 studies reported events such as cough, dizziness, diarrhoea, low blood sugar, gastrointestinal upset, headache, epigastric distension, dry mouth, skin itching, urticaria, heart palpitations. Liver biochemistry was abnormal in five cases after treatment and hyperkalaemia was reported in one patient after control.	

The risk in the intervention group (and its 95% CI) is based on the assumed risk in the comparison group and the relative effect of the intervention (and its 95% CI).

[1] Unclear sequence generation and allocation concealment. Lack of blinding of participants and personnel.
[2] Wide CI and small sample size,
[3] Wide CI,
[4] Considerable statistical heterogeneity.

Abbreviations: ACEi, angiotensin-converting enzyme inhibitor; ACR, albumin lo creatinine ratio: ARB, angiotensin-receptor blockers; CHM, Chinese herbal medicine; CI, confidence interval; CT, conventional treatments; eGFR: estimated glomerular filtration rate; ESRD: end-stage renal disease; MD: mean difference; RCTs: randomised controlled trial, RR, risk ratio; SCr: serum creatinine; Td: treatment duration.

Study References: All-cause mortality, Progression to ESRD, and albuminuria progression: H10; eGFR: H5, H21–H38; SCr: H4, H9, H11, H21, H23–H25, H27, H29–H31, H33–H35, H63, H69, H72–H160; Albuminuria: H23, H31, H37, H72, H87, H98, H141, H146, H235–H242; Adverse events: H8, H10, H23–H25, H33, H72, H75, H81, H85–H87, H89, H90, H92–H94, H96, H102, H105, H106, HI09, H117–H121, H123, H125, H127, H130, HI32, H134, H135, H137, H138, H235, H249, H250, H253, H254, H256, H257, H262, H264, H270, H284, H287, H291, H292, H294, H295, H297, H299, H302, H304, H306, H308–H310, H312, H313, H316, H317, H322, H343, H346, H348, H352, H398, H404, H405, H408, H420, H424, H425, H142, H143, H146–H148, H150, H274, H275, H326, H422, H152, H154, H155, H160, H276, H277, H280, H281, H330, H333, H334, H336–H338.

Table 5.14.   GRADE: Oral Chinese Herbal Medicine Plus Conventional Treatment vs. Conventional Treatment Plus ACEi/ARB

Outcomes	GRADE	Anticipated Absolute Effects	
		Risk with CTs and ACEi/ARB	**Risk Difference with CHM and CTs**
All-cause mortality, progression to ESRD, and change in CKD stage			Not measured
eGFR-Cockcroft-Gault Td: mean 10 weeks N = 171(2RCTs)	⊕○○○ VERY LOW[1,2,3]	The mean eGFR was 98.51 mL/min	MD 1.35 mL/min lower (17.16 lower to 14.45 higher)
SCr Td: mean 10.76 weeks N = 1,580 (21 RCTs)	⊕⊕○○ LOW[1,3]	The mean SCr was 83.32 µmol/L	MD 0.10 µmol/L lower (2.06 lower to 1.86 higher)
Albuminuria Assessed with: ACR Td: mean 10.67 weeks N = 196(3RCTs)	⊕⊕○○ LOW[1,4]	The mean ACR was 127.01 mg/g	MD 28.84 mg/g lower (36.89 lower to 20.78 lower)

(Continued)

Table 5.14. (*Continued*)

		Anticipated Absolute Effects	
Outcomes	GRADE	Risk with CTs and ACEi/ARB	Risk Difference with CHM and CTs
All-cause mortality, progression to ESRD, and change in CKD stage		Not measured	
Adverse events N = 1,836 (27 RCTs)		A total of 14 studies reported that no adverse events occurred. A total of 13 studies reported the following adverse events in a small number of participants: dry mouth, dry cough, hypoglycaemia, dizziness, hypotension in the control group. Diarrhoea, abdominal discomfort, nausea, loose stools, dark/black stools, hypoglycaemia in the treatment group.	

The risk in the intervention group (and its 95% CI) is based on the assumed risk in the comparison group and the relative effect of the intervention (and its 95% CI). 1. Unclear sequence generation and allocation concealment. Lack of blinding of participants and personnel. 2. Wide confidence interval and small sample size. 3. Considerable statistical heterogeneity. 4. Small sample size.

Abbreviations: ACEi, angiotensin-converting enzyme inhibitor; ACR. albumin to creatinine ratio; ARB, angiotensin-receptor blockers; CHM, Chinese herbal medicine; CI, confidence interval; CKD, chronic kidney disease; CT. conventional treatments; eGFR, estimated glomerular filtration rate; ESRD: end-stage renal disease; MD, mean difference; RCTs: randomised controlled trial; SCr, serum creatinine; Td, treatment duration.

Study References: eGFR: H39, H40; SCr: H39, H40, H46, H63, H69, H73, H128, H140, H143, H147, H161–H163, H164, H165, H166, H167, H168–H171; Albuminuria: H379, H418, H437; Adverse events: H40, H70, H71, H143, H147, H162, H164, H165, H167, H169, H170, H183, H253, H309, H356, H361, H367, H371, H373, H378, H379, M382, H384, H387, H390, H391.

5. *Oral CHM Plus CT Plus ACEi Placebo vs. Placebo CHM Plus CT Plus ACEi*

Evidence from one study which compared oral CHM to ACEi with double dummy design was low quality (Table 5.15). Compared to ACEi, eGFR was higher and albuminuria excretion was lower in the CHM plus CT group (low certainty evidence).

Table 5.15   GRADE: Chinese Herbal Medicine Plus Conventional Treatment Plus ACEi/ARB Placebo vs. Chinese Herbal Medicine Placebo Plus Conventional Treatment Plus ACEi/ARBs

		Anticipated Absolute Effects	
Outcomes	**GRADE**	**Risk with CTs and ACEi/ARB and CHM Placebo**	**Risk Difference with CHM and CTs and ACEi/ARB Placebo**
eGFR-Cockcroft-Gault Td: 8 weeks N = 90 (1 RCTs)	⊕⊕○○ LOW[1,2]	The mean eGFR was 112.83 mL/min	MD 9.99 mL/min lower (13.62 lower to 6.36 lower)
SCr Td: 8 weeks N = 90 (1 RCTs)	⊕⊕○○ LOW[1,2]	The mean SCr was 88.67 µmol/L	MD 2.04 µmol/L lower (6.29 lower to 2.21 higher)
Albuminuria Assessed with: AER Td: 8 weeks N = 90 (1 RCTs)	⊕⊕○○ LOW[1,2]	The mean AER was 84.72 mg/24h	MD 44.55 mg/24h lower (47.03 lower to 42.07 lower)
Adverse events		Not reported	

The risk in the intervention group (and its 95% CI) is based on the assumed risk in the comparison group and the relative effect of the intervention (and its 95% CI). 1. Unclear sequence generation and allocation concealment. 2. Small sample size.

Abbreviations: ACEi, angiotensin-converting enzyme inhibitor; AER, albumin excretion rate; ARB, angiotensin-receptor blockers; CHM, Chinese herbal medicine; CI, confidence interval; CT, conventional treatments; eGFR, estimated glomerular filtration rate; MD, mean difference; RCTs, randomised controlled trial; SCr, serum creatinine; Td. treatment duration.

Study References: eGFR, SCr: and Albuminuria: H41

Randomised Controlled Trial Evidence for Individual Oral Formulae

Most of the formulae tested in the included studies were similar but not identical. This may have led to heterogeneity among studies, given that 11 individual oral formulae, including commercial products, were tested in multiple trials. The analysis results of these individual formulae are presented in Table 5.16, and summarised as follows.

Dong chong xia cao preparation

Dong chong xia cao 冬虫夏草制剂 preparation was made of fermented *Cordyceps sinensis* (Berk.) Sacc powder. It was in the form of a manufactured capsule with three different commercial brands (*Bai ling capsule* 百令胶囊, *Jin shui bao capsule* 金水宝胶囊 and *Zhi ling* capsule 至灵胶囊).

- Compared to CTs, *Dong chong xia cao* preparation plus CTs reduced SCr concentration but did not produce additional benefit with respect to reducing albuminuria at the end of treatment (four to eight weeks) in type 2 diabetes patients with microalbuminuria (low quality evidence).
- Compared to ACEi or ARBs, the combination of *Dong chong xia cao* preparation and ACEi or ARBs did not show further benefit for either eGFR (estimated by Cockcroft-Gault equation) or SCr after three months of treatment, but reduced SCr concentration with a longer treatment duration (≥ three months). The combination reduced ACR (very low to low quality evidence). The combination showed a more pronounced reduction of blood lipids (TC, TG and LDL), but not blood glucose or BP (not graded).

Bu yang huan wu tang

Bu yang huan wu tang 补阳还五汤 is comprised of *huang qi* 黄芪, *dang gui* 当归, *chi shao* 赤芍, *di long* 地龙, *chuang xiong* 川芎, *hong hua* 红花 and *tao ren* 桃仁. *Bu yang huan wu tang* appeared to reduce albuminuria.

Table 5.16. Individual Formula Results

Intervention	Comparator	No. of Studies (Duration)	No. of Participants	Outcome (Unit)	Effect Size MD [95% CI]	I²	GRADE	Included Studies
Dong chong xia cao preparation 冬虫夏草制剂 + CT	CT	2 (4–8w)	140	SCr (μmol/L)	−9.20 [−14.14, −4.25]*	0%	Low[1,2]	H42, H69
		1 (4w)	80	AER (mg/24h)	−1.60 [−8.67, 5.47]	NA	Low[1,2]	H42
Dong chong xia cao preparation 冬虫夏草制剂 + CT + ACEi/ARBs	CT + ACEi/ARBs	4 (4w–12m)	304	eGFR(mL/min)	−6.88 [−18.67, 4.91]	79.4%	Very low[1,2,3]	H24, H28, H36, H37
		14 (4w–6m)	1,040	SCr (μmol/L)	−3.68 [−8.14, 0.79]	81.8%	Low[1,3]	H24, H69, H75, H80, H83, H96, H100, H105, H112, H114, H118, H119, H145, H149
		3 (6–12w)	208	ACR (mg/g)	−16.46 [−24.84, −8.07]*	47.6%	Low[1,2]	H37, H240, H241
Bu yang huan wu tang (modified) 补阳还五汤加减 + CT	CT	3 (4–12w)	188	AER (μg/min)	−69.38 [−137.84, −0.92]*	99.6%	Very low[1,2,3]	H44, H211, H214
Bu yang huan wu tang (modified) 补阳还五汤加减 + CT + ACEi	CT + ACEi	2 (4–12w)	144	AER (mg/24h)	−12.90[−18.86, −6.93]*	0%	Low[1,2]	H88, H255
Liu wei di huang wan (modified) 六味地黄丸(加减) + CT	CT + ACEi/ARBs	2 (12w)	128	AER (μg/min)	−32.99 [−52.51, −13.47]*	75%	Very low[1,2,3]	H376, H389

(Continued)

Table 5.16. (*Continued*)

Intervention	Comparator	No. of Studies (Duration)	No. of Participants	Outcome (Unit)	Effect Size MD [95% CI]	I^2	GRADE	Included Studies
Liu wei di huang wan (modified) 六味地黄丸(加减) + CT + ACEi	CT + ACEi	2 (8w)	180	AER (mg/24h)	−32.12 [−64.58, 0.35]	96%	Very low[1,2,3]	H305, H336
Jin gui shen qi wan 金匮肾气丸 + CT + ACEi	CT + ACEi	1 (2m)	60	SCr (μmol/L)	−11.70 [−17.95, −5.45]*	NA	Low[1,2]	H104
		2 (1–2m)	130	AER (μg/min)	−27.02 [−55.51, 1.48]	96.0%	Very low[1,2,3]	H105, H327
Shen qi di huang tang (modified) 参芪地黄汤(加味) + CT + ACEi/ARBs	CT + ACEi/ARBs	1 (8w)	98	SCr (μmol/L)	−3.10 [−4.25, −1.95]*	NA	Low[1,2]	H91
		1 (8w)	68	AER (mg/24h)	−26.37 [−49.10, −3.64]*	NA	Low[1,2]	H246
Niao du qing granule 尿毒清颗粒 + CT	CT	2 (3m)	146	SCr (μmol/L)	−7.40 [−10.75, −4.04]*	0.0%	Low[1,2]	H52, H56
		3 (3–6m)	226	AER (μg/min)	−56.36 [−84.57, −28.16]*	87.5%	Very low[1,2,3]	H18, H52, H56
Shen yan kang fu pian 肾炎康复片 + CT	CT	2 (12w)	104	AER (mg/24h)	−34.45 [−43.06, −25.85]*	0%	Low[1,2]	H70, H71
Shen yan kang fu pian 肾炎康复片 + CT	CT + ARBs	2 (12w)	105	AER (mg/24h)	−8.23 [−17.96, 1.49]	23%	Low[1,2]	H70, H71
Huang kui capsule 黄葵胶囊 + CT	CT	2 (8–12w)	152	AER (μg/min)	−33.05 [−47.77, −18.33]*	78.5%	Very low[1,2,3]	H51, H219

Formula	Intervention	No. of studies (duration)	No. of participants	Outcome	MD [95%CI]	I^2	Certainty	Included studies
Huang kui capsule 黄葵胶囊 + CT + ARBs	CT + ARBs	1 (16w)	65	eGFR(mL/min)	0.30 [−11.94, 12.54]	NA	Low[1,2]	H34
		2 (6–16w)	160	SCr (μmol/L)	−0.76 [−5.11, 3.60]	0.0%	Low[1,2]	H34, H109
		2 (6–16w)	160	AER (μg/min)	−16.82 [−38.28, 4.64]	96.0%	Very low[1,2,3]	H34, H109
Qi shen yi qi di wan 芪参益气滴丸 + CT + ACEi	CT + ACEi	1 (12w)	60	SCr (μmol/L)	−1.61 [−12.08, 8.86]	NA	Low[1,2]	H4
		2 (8–12w)	122	AER (μg/min)	−41.83 [−56.27, −27.40]*	44.9%	Low[1,2]	H4, H288
Zhi dan jiang tang capsule 丹蛭降糖胶囊 + CT + ACEi/ARBs	CT + ACEi/ ARBs	2 (8w)	129	AER (μg/min)	−26.50 [−30.30, −22.71]*	24.6%	Low[1,2]	H291, H310
Tong xin luo capsule 通心络胶囊 + CT + ACEi/ARBs	CT + ACEi/ ARBs	3 (8–24w)	206	SCr (μmol/L)	−2.84 [−7.19, 1.50]	38.3%	Low[1,2]	H21, H124, H133
		3 (8–24w)	174	AER (μg/min)	−22.62 [−42.43, −2.81]*	85.8%	Very low[1,2,3]	H21, H124, H296
Fu fang xue shuan tong capsule 复方血栓通胶囊 + CT + ACEi/ARBs	CT + ACEi/ ARBs	2 (3–6m)	138	SCr (μmol/L)	−17.14 [−29.78, −4.49]*	86.6%	Very low[1,2,3]	H117, H134
		1 (6m)	120	ACR (mg/g)	−22.88 [−34.86, −10.90]*	NA	Low[1,2]	H239

Notes: Formula was selected if there were two or more studies using the same formula.

Abbreviations: 95%CI, 95% confidence interval; ACEi, angiotensin-converting enzyme inhibitor; ACR, albumin to creatinine ratio; AER, albumin excretion rate; ARB, angiotensin-receptor blockers; CT, conventional treatment; eGFR, estimated glomerular filtration rate; MD, mean difference; NA, not applicable; SCr, serum creatinine.

#eGFR was estimated by Cockcroft-Gault equation.
*Statistically significant.

1. Unclear sequence generation and allocation concealment. Lack of blinding for participants and personnel.
2. Small sample size limited certainty of results.
3. Considerable statistical heterogeneity.

- Compared to CTs, *Bu yang huan wu tang* 补阳还五汤 plus CTs reduced AER at the end of the treatment (four weeks to three months) (very low quality evidence).
- Compared to ACEi, combination of *Bu yang huan wu tang* and ACEi may reduce AER at the end of four to 12 weeks treatment (low quality evidence).

Liu wei di huang wan

Liu wei di huang wan 六味地黄丸 contains *di huang* 地黄, *shan zhu yu* 山茱萸, *shan yao* 山药, *fu ling* 茯苓, *mu dan pi* 牡丹皮, and *ze xie* 泽泻. *Liu wei di huang wan* did not show a conclusive result with respect to albuminuria reduction (very low quality evidence).

- Compared to ACEi or ARBs, results from two RCTs showed that AER was reduced by treatment with *Liu wei di huang wan* for four to 12 weeks. Two other RCTs evaluated antiproteinuric effects did not show a significant difference between *Liu wei di huang wan* plus ACEi and ACEi alone.

Jin gui shen qi wan

The ingredients of *Jin gui shen qi wan* 金匮肾气丸 are similar to *Liu wei di huang wan* 六味地黄丸. In addition to the six ingredients in *Liu wei di huang wan*, it also contains *gui zhi* 桂枝 and *fu zi* 附子.

- The limited number of trials that tested the clinical effects of *Jin gui shen qi wan* 金匮肾气丸 combined with ACEi did not show an additional benefit for albuminuria reduction (very low quality evidence).

Shen qi di huang tang

Shen qi di huang tang 参芪地黄汤 is comprised of *ren shen* 人参, *huang qi* 黄芪, *shu di huang* 地黄, *shan zhu yu* 山茱萸, *shan yao* 山药, *mu dan pi* 牡丹皮, *sheng jiang* 生姜, *da zao* 大枣.

- Three RCTs evaluated the clinical effects of *Shen qi di huang tang*. Compared to ACEi or ARBs, *Shen qi di huang tang* plus ACEi or ARBs reduced SCr and albuminuria (in terms of AER and UAC) (low quality evidence), and resulted in further reductions in HbA1c and blood lipids (TC and TG), but not in BP (not graded).

Niao du qing granule

Niao du qing granule 尿毒清颗粒 is a commercial product which contains *da huang* 大黄, *huang qi* 黄芪, *sang bai pi* 桑白皮, *ku shen* 苦参, *bai zhu* 白术, *he shou wu* 何首乌, *bai shao* 白芍, *dan shen* 丹参 and *che qian cao*车前草.

- Compared to CTs, SCr and albuminuria were decreased with the treatment of *Niao du qing* granule for three to six months (very low to low quality evidence).

Shen yan kang fu pian

Shen yan kang fu pian 肾炎康复片 is a commercial product which contains *xi yang shen* 西洋参, *ren shen* 人参, *di huang* 地黄, *du zhong* 杜仲, *shan yao* 山药, *bai hua she she cao* 白花蛇舌草, *tu fu ling* 土茯苓, *yi mu cao* 益母草, *dan shen* 丹参, *ze xie* 泽泻, *bai mao gen* 白茅根, *jie geng* 桔梗 and *hei dou* 黑豆.

- *Shen yan kang fu pian* may reduce AER compared to CTs, but there was no significant difference when compared to ARB (low quality evidence).

Huang kui capsule

Huang kui capsule 黄葵胶囊 is a commercial product which is made of *Abelmoschus Manihot* (L.) Medic. Flower. (*Huang Shu Kui hua*)

- Compared to CTs, *Huang kui* capsule 黄葵胶囊 plus CT reduced AER after eight to 12 week treatment (very low quality evidence).
- Adding *Huang kui* capsule to ARBs may improve AER and UPE compared to ARBs after six to 16 weeks of treatment, but there was no significant difference in eGFR and SCr (very low to low quality evidence).

Qi shen yi qi di wan

Qi shen yi qi di wan 芪参益气滴丸 (dripping pill) is a commercial product which contains *huang qi* 黄芪, *dan shen* 丹参, *san qi* 三七 and *jiang xiang you* 降香油.

- At the end of treatment (eight to 12 weeks), the combination of *Qi shen yi qi di wan* and ARBs reduced AER but not SCr compared to ARBs (low quality evidence).

Zhi dan jiang tang capsule

Zhi dan jiang tang capsule 丹蛭降糖胶囊 is comprised of *mu dan pi* 牡丹皮, *di huang* 地黄, *ze xie* 泽泻, *tai zi shen* 太子参, *tu si zi* 菟丝子, etc.

- Added to ACEi or ARBs over eight weeks treatment may reduce AER (low quality evidence).

Tong xin luo capsule

Tong xin luo capsule 通心络胶囊 is a commercial product which contains *ren shen* 人参, *shui zhi* 水蛭, *quan xie* 全蝎, *chi shao* 赤芍, *chan tui* 蝉蜕, *tu bie chong* 土鳖虫, *wu gong* 蜈蚣, *tan xiang* 檀香, *jiang xiang* 降香, *ru xiang* 乳香, *suan zao ren* 酸枣仁 and *bing pian* 冰片.

- Added to ACEi or ARBs over eight to 24 weeks treatment may reduce AER but not SCr (very low to low quality evidence).

Fu fang xue shuan tong capsule

Fu fang xue shuan tong capsule 复方血栓通胶囊 is a commercial product which is comprised of *san qi* 三七, *huang qi* 黄芪, *dan shen* 丹参 and *xuan shen* 玄参.

- At the end of three to six months of treatment, *Fu fang xue shuan tong* capsule plus ACEi or ARBs may further reduce SCr but not blood glucose, BP and lipid compared to ACEi or ARBs (low quality evidence).
- Based on evidence from a single RCT, the combination may reduce UPE and albuminuria in terms of ACR, AER and UAC (very low quality evidence).

Clinical Evidence for Commonly Used Chinese Herbal Medicine Treatments

Several different CHM were recommended by the CM clinical practice guidelines and text books, which were mostly based on experts' consensus (refer to Chapter 2). In this chapter, we identified clinical trials evaluating the efficacy and safety of some of these recommended formulae. Therefore, the clinical evidence underpinning the use of the guideline recommended CHM treatments are summarised.

Dong chong xia cao preparation 冬虫夏草制剂, which was made of fermented *Cordyceps sinensis* (Berk.) Sacc powder, was the most frequently studied CHM intervention. Twenty-nine RCTs researched the add-on effect of *Dong chong xia cao* preparation in people with DKD. They found that *Dong chong xia cao* preparation showed extra benefit in reducing SCr concentration and albuminuria excretion when used in combination with pharmacotherapy. However, the quality of the evidence was low. Another manufactured CHM product mentioned in guidelines and identified in clinical evidence was *Huang kui* capsule 黄葵胶囊. There were four RCTs and a case series study which used the *Huang kui* capsule (*Abelmoschus Manihot* (L.) Medic. Flower) as intervention. Proteinuria and albuminuria excretion were lower with treatment than control. However, the low quality evidence substantially reduced the confidence in the beneficial effect demonstrated by *Huang kui* capsule.

As for oral decoction, both *Jin gui shen qi wan* 金匮肾气丸 and *Shen qi di huang tang* 参芪地黄汤 were recommended in different text books and CM guidelines. Only two RCTs of *Jin gui shen qi wan* and four RCTs of *Shen qi di huang tang* were found eligible for meta-analysis. Pool estimates of the effect of *Jin gui shen qi wan* from two RCTs did not show an additional advantage for albuminuria reduction when used in combination with ACEi. For *Shen qi di huang tang*, individual RCTs measuring the outcomes of SCr and albuminuria favoured combination with ACEi or ARBs compared with either agent alone.

Frequently Reported Orally Used Herbs in Meta-analyses Showing Favourable Effects

In order to identify the most promising herbal candidates for treatment of DKD and future research, the frequencies of herbs used in studies that were identified in the meta-analyses showing a favourable effect were calculated. The herbal frequency was analysed based on different outcome categories. The kidney function category con-

Table 5.17. Frequently Reported Herbs in Meta-Analyses Showing Favourable Effect

Herbs	Scientific Name
Huang qi 黄芪	*Astragalus membranaceus* (Fisch.) Bge.
Dan shen 丹参	*Salvia miltiorrhiza* Bge.
(Shu) di huang (熟)地黄	*Rehmannia glutinosa* Libosch.
Shan yao 山药	*Dioscorea opposita* Thunb.
Chuan xiong 川芎	*Ligusticum chuanxiong* Hort.
Fu ling 茯苓	*Poria cocos* (Schw.) Wolf
Shan zhu yu 山茱萸	*Cornus officinalis* Sieb. & Zucc.
Dang gui 当归	*Angelica sinensis (Oliv.)* Diels
Da huang 大黄	*Rheum palmatum* L.; *Rheum tanguticum* Maxim. Ex Balf.; *Rheum officinale* Baill.
Ze xie 泽泻	*Alisma orientalis* (Sam.) Juzep.; *Alisma plantago-aquatica* L.

Outcomes included kidney function, albuminuira, and proteinuria. Kidney function: refer to Table 5.5 and 5.6; Albuminuria and Proteinuria refer to Table 5.8, 5.9 and 5.10.

sisted of meta-analyses of outcomes of GFR, eGFR or serum creatinine, in which the pool estimated results favoured the CHM groups. The categories of albuminuria and proteinuria were analysed according to the same method, including meta-analyses favouring the CHM groups regardless of comparators.

The top ten most common herbs of the meta-analyses favouring the use of CHM are listed in Table 5.17. The top ten herbs were identical among the three different outcome categories, but the ranking of each herb was slightly different. Among the three outcome categories, *huang qi* 黄芪 was the most common, followed by *dan shen* 丹参, *di huang* 地黄 and *shan yao* 山药.

Non-randomised Controlled Clinical Trials of Oral Chinese Herbal Medicine

Three CCTs evaluated the effects of CHM in patients with DKD (H438–H440). These CCTs allocated participants without randomisation and therefore differed from RCTs. The three included CCTs were all conducted in China, involving 246 participants. Two studies included patients with kidney disease caused by type 2 diabetes (H438, H439), while the other trial did not clearly state this parameter (H440). The included participants were aged from 33 to 81 years, and the mean age was 57 years. Treatment duration ranged from six weeks to three months.

All three studies administered oral CHM in addition to ACEi/ARB. ACEi were used in both the intervention and control groups in two studies (H438, H440), while ARB was used in one (H439). The CHM formulae tested in the three studies were different and included *Shen qi jiang tang granule* 参芪降糖颗粒, *Yin xing ye pill* 银杏叶片 and *Yi shen tang* 益肾汤. The herbal ingredients used in more than two studies were *di huang* 地黄, *huang qi* 黄芪 and *wu wei zi* 五味子.

The pooled estimate of two studies showed the effect of CHM as an adjunct to ACEi and CTs on SCr was uncertain (MD −0.67μmol/L [−6.40, 5.06], I² = 0%) (H438, H440). However, both the meta-analysis and single study results favoured the combination use of CHM with ACEi or ARB in reducing albuminuria and proteinuria (Table 5.18). All studies did not report any adverse events during the study period.

Non-controlled Studies of Oral Chinese Herbal Medicine

Twenty-four non-controlled studies were assessed, including three case reports and 21 case series (H441–H464). The total number of participants with DKD was 1,174, of whom 861 were reported to have type 2 diabetes. Among the eight studies which provided information regarding CM syndrome, *qi* and *yin* deficiency with Blood stasis and Spleen and/or Kidney deficiency were the most common syndromes (three studies).

Most of the studies applied self-prescribed formulae, except for five studies which prescribed manufactured CM medicines (H443, H447, H448, H457, H458). Eight studies (H447, H448, H451, H453, H454, H458–H460) used CHM added to ACEi/ARB and CTs, while the other 16 studies did not apply ACEi or ARB. Treatment duration ranged from four weeks to six months, and the mode duration was two months.

Among the 24 studies, 23 distinct formulae were identified. The manufactured medicine *Tong xin luo capsule* 通心络胶囊 appeared

Table 5.18. Oral Chinese Herbal Medicine Plus ACEi/ARBs Plus Conventional Treatment vs. ACEi/ARBs Plus Conventional Treatment (Controlled Clinical Trials)

Outcome (Unit)	No. of Studies	No. of Participants	MD [95% CI]	I^2%	Included Studies
eGFR (mL/min)	1	86	1.80 [−1.41, 5.01]	NA	H439
SCr (μmol/L)	2	160	−0.67 [−6.40, 5.06]	0%	H438, H440
AER (μg/min)	2	206	−20.56 [−32.96, −8.16]*	48%	H439, H440
AER (mg/24h)	1	40	−43.82 [−75.17, −12.47]*	NA	H438
UPE (g/24h)	1	86	−0.04 [−0.06, −0.02]*	NA	H439
FBG (mmol/L)	3	246	−0.17 [−0.52, 0.18]	0%	H438–H440
HbA1c (%)	1	40	−0.01 [−0.19, 0.17]	NA	H438
TC (mmol/L)	1	40	0.04 [−0.57, 0.65]	NA	H438
TG (mmol/L)	1	40	−0.02 [−0.18, 0.14]	NA	H438

*Statistically significant.

Abbreviations: AER, albumin excretion rate; eGFR: estimated glomerular filtration rate; HbA1c, haemoglobinA1c; FBG, fasting blood glucose; NA: not applicable, SCr, serum creatinine; TC, total cholesterol; TG, total glucose; UPE, urinary protein excretion.

twice in different studies (H447, H448). Its composition included *ren shen* 人参, *shui zhi* 水蛭, *wu gong* 蜈蚣, *tu bie chong* 土鳖虫, *quan xie* 全蝎 and *chi shao* 赤芍, and is indicated for Blood activation. As for the commonly reported herbs, *di huang* 地黄, *huang qi* 黄芪 and *shan zhu yu* 山茱萸 were the top three with frequencies in excess of 10 (Table 5.19). In general, the frequently used herbs were those with tonifying and replenishing, Blood-activating, dampness-draining, heat-clearing and astringent properties.

Studies of Oral Plus Rectal (Enema) Chinese Herbal Medicine

One RCT (H1) evaluated the effects of oral combined with rectal CHM for early DKD. The study enrolled 80 participants aged from 44

Table 5.19. Frequently Reported Herbs in Non-controlled Studies

Most Common Herbs	Scientific Name	Frequency of Use
Di huang 地黄	*Rehmannia glutinosa* Libosch.	17
Huang qi 黄芪	*Astragalus membranaceus* (Fisch.) Bge.	15
Shan zhu yu 山茱萸	*Cornus officinalis* Sieb. & Zucc.	11
Dan shen 丹参	*Salvia miltiorrhiza* Bge.	9
Gou qi zi 枸杞子	*Lycium barbarum* L.	9
Shan yao 山药	*Dioscorea opposita* Thunb.	8
Chi shao 赤芍	*Paeonia lactiflora* Pall.	6
Chuan xiong 川芎	*Ligusticum chuanxiong* Hort.	6
Fu ling 茯苓	*Poria cocos* (Schw.) Wolf	6
Bai zhu 白术	*Atractylodes macrocephala* Koidz.	5
Dang gui 当归	*Angelica sinensis* (Oliv.) Diels	5
Mai dong 麦冬	*Ophiopogon japonicus* Ker.-Gawl.	5
Tai zi shen 太子参	*Pseudostellaria heterophylla* (Miq.) Pax ex Pax et Hoffm.	5
Xuan shen 玄参	*Scrophularia ningpoensis* Hemsl.	5
Huang lian 黄连	*Coptis chinensis* Franch.	4
Niu xi 牛膝	*Achyranthes bidentata* Bl.	4
Tian hua fen 天花粉	*Tirchosanthes kirilowii* Maxim.	4
Wu wei zi 五味子	*Schisandra chinensis* (Turcz.) Baill.	4
Xu duan 续断	*Dipsacus asper* Wall.	4
Ze xie 泽泻	*Alisma orientalis* (Sam.) Juzep.	4

Note: The use of some herbs may be restricted in some countries; readers are advised to comply with relevant regulations.

to 73 years old and diagnosed with *qi* and *yin* deficiency with Blood stasis. All participants received CTs (including dietary and exercise advice, blood glucose and lipid control) and ramipril. *Yi qi yang yin huo xue tang* 益气养阴活血汤 was orally administered twice daily and CHM retention enema was administered once daily for approximately 30 minutes. Treatments lasted for three months. *Yi qi yang yin huo xue tang* 益气养阴活血汤 contained *huang qi* 黄芪, *dan shen* 丹

参, *xuan shen* 玄参, *huang jing* 黄精, *di huang* 地黄, *shan zhu yu* 山茱萸, *mai dong* 麦冬, *dang gui* 当归, *shan yao* 山药, *gou qi zi* 枸杞子, *chi shao* 赤芍 and *wu wei zi* 五味子. The herb ingredients of CHM enema formula differed from oral formula except for *dan shen* 丹参. It contained *da huang* 大黄, *mu li* 牡蛎, *fu zi* 附子, *dan shen* 丹参, *huai hua* 槐花, *ze xie* 泽泻, and *huang qin* 黄芩.

Risk of Bias

The study was described as "randomised", but neither the method for sequence generation nor information on allocation concealment was mentioned. Participants and personnel and outcome assessors were not blinded. Outcome data were complete and there were no missing data or drop-outs. Selective outcome reporting was at unclear risk of bias because the study protocol was not available. Overall, the methodological quality of the study was very low.

Outcomes

The results showed that the CHM combination treatments produced additional benefit on AER (MD −23.29μg/min [−39.27, −7.31]) and SCr (MD −10.99μmol/L [−16.85, −5.13]) reduction. FBG decreased in both groups after treatments, but there was no difference between groups (MD −0.25mmol/L [−0.58, 0.08]. The effect on blood lipid regulation was uncertain: TC (MD −0.65mmol/L [−1.59, 0.29]), TG (MD −0.60mmol/L [−1.15, −0.05]), LDL (MD −0.84mmol/L [−1.22, −0.46]), HDL (0.17mmol/L [0.01, 0.33]).

The study did not report whether any adverse events occurred during the research period. Therefore, the safety of oral plus rectal CHM for patients with DKD is uncertain.

Safety of Chinese Herbal Medicine Treatments for Diabetic Kidney Disease

Among the 464 included studies (RCTs, CCTs and non-controlled studies), 165 studies (36%) involving 11,716 participants reported safety outcomes. The majority of these studies reported that no adverse events occurred during the study periods. In total, 166 adverse events (AEs) were observed in 44 studies with a sample size of 3,194 participants. Six studies only reported clinical manifestations of AEs without exact numbers of cases or cases in each group. The number of AEs observed in participants who received CHM treatment was 88. In RCTs, 81 cases of AEs were observed in the CHM group while 74 cases were found in the control groups (Table 5.20). With CHM treatments, the most common AEs were digestive upset, such as diarrhoea, loose stool, loss of appetite and upper abdominal discomfort. There were seven cases of withdrawal in the CHM groups due to intolerance related to diarrhoea. Furthermore, cases of dry cough caused by ACEi were less common when combined with CHM.

In the non-controlled studies, nine studies reported information of AEs among the 572 participants. Of these, six studies stated that no AEs were observed. Another three studies reported five cases of upper abdominal upset and two cases of dry cough. The digestive discomforts were relieved by taking medicine after meals, and dry cough was resolved by replacing captopril with valsartan. None of the participants were withdrawn due to AEs.

Table 5.20. Adverse Events in Randomised Controlled Trials

Adverse Events	CHM Group (n)	Control Group (n)
Digestive upset	61	6
Dry cough	10	39
Hypoglycaemia	3	8
Hypotension	0	4
Hyperkalaemia	0	2
Dizziness or headache	6	12
Elevated transaminase level	1	0
Skin itching or urticaria	0	2
Dry mouth	0	1
Total	81	74

Summary of Chinese Herbal Medicine Clinical Evidence

Chinese herbal medicine has been widely used in clinical CM practice for treating symptoms associated with DKD. Following comprehensive searching, more than five thousand studies were identified and 464 were eligible for further analysis. All included studies used CHM as integrative medicine with CTs prescribed according to the management recommendations of international clinical practice guidelines. Among the included studies, CHM was administered orally in all except one study. There was no fixed treatment course for CHM, and the treatment durations ranged from two weeks to two years.

Chinese Medicine Syndrome Differentiation

Information of CM syndrome differentiation was mentioned in 185 studies (40%). After standardisation, *qi* and/or *yin* deficiency with Blood stasis was the most common syndrome. This finding was consistent with the effects of the high frequency herbs. Among all included studies, whether or not CM syndromes formed part of the inclusion criteria, the top three herbs were *huang qi* 黄芪, *di huang* 地黄 and *dan shen* 丹参. These were typically prescribed to tonify *qi*, replenish *yin* and activate Blood according to CM theory. These results suggest that *qi* and/or *yin* deficiency with Blood stasis may be the core syndrome for patients with early stage DKD.

Formulae and Herbs

Nearly 364 distinct formulae with over two hundred kinds of herbs were identified from eligible studies. CHM was administered in the form of decoctions, granules, capsules, tablets or pills. Some of the formulae with fixed compositions or specific active components had been developed as manufactured products. For example, the most common single-herb formula, *Dong chong xia cao* preparation 冬虫

夏草制剂, originated from fermented *Cordyceps sinensis* and was then processed as commercial capsules. Though some formulae were unnamed and some were self-titled, by checking the ingredients, it appeared that *Liu wei di huang wan* 六味地黄丸 was the core formula across studies and formulae used in many trials were modified based on its composition.

Some formulae were common and appeared across different types of studies. For example, *Tong xin luo capsule* 通心络胶囊 was assessed in five RCTs and two non-controlled studies; *Huang kui capsule* 黄葵胶囊 was used in four RCTs and one non-controlled study; and *Yin xing ye* preparation 银杏叶制剂 was tested in three RCTs and one CCT. Meta-analysis of RCTs favoured combination use of *Tong xin luo capsule* 通心络胶囊 or *Huang kui capsule* 黄葵胶囊 with CTs and reduced urinary albumin excretion, but the quality of evidence was very low to low.

Overall Evidence

The majority of studies evaluated the effects of CHM on patients with DKD and microalbuminuria by examining the outcomes of GFR (or eGFR), SCr, urinary albumin or protein excretion, and other laboratory biomarkers related to kidney injury and diabetes.

It was uncertain whether CHM in combination with ACEi/ARB and CTs was able to reduce mortality and progression to ESRD (defined as commencement of dialysis). It was also uncertain whether orally administered CHM combined with CT was able to lower urinary albumin and protein excretion because the certainty of the evidence was very low. However, when combined with ACEi/ARB and CTs, CHM may further lower urinary albumin and protein excretion. Adding CHM to CTs may also reduce SCr concentration regardless of combined use with ACEi/ARB. CHM, when combined with CTs, may decrease SCr concentration in early stage DKD (eGFR > 60mL/min), and longer treatment durations may produce a more beneficial effect. When combined with ACEi/ARB, CHM decreased SCr concentration in populations with advanced

DKD (eGFR ≤ 60mL/min), although the certainty of this evidence was low. There was no compelling evidence showing that CHM can improve eGFR.

Blood pressure was reduced by both CHM alone and ACEi/ARB alone, but the reduction was greater with ACEi/ARB compared to CHM. Compared to controls, neither CHM in combination with CTs nor in combination with ACEi/ARBs showed additional benefit on BP. There was no difference between CHM added to hypoglycaemic agents and hypoglycaemic agents alone. CHM showed a positive effect on regulation of dyslipidaemia, whether used alone or in conjunction with lipid-lowering agents.

As for the effects of individual formulae, *Bu yang huan wu tang* (modified) 补阳还五汤加减, *Niao du qing* granule 尿毒清颗粒, *Shen yan kang fu pian* 肾炎康复片 and *Huang kui* capsule 黄葵胶囊 were found to reduce albuminuria when used as integrated therapy. *Dong chong xia cao* preparations 冬虫夏草制剂 and *Niao du qing* granule in conjunction with CTs lowered SCr concentration.

When combined with ACEi/ARB, *Dong chong xia cao* preparation 冬虫夏草制剂, *Bu yang huan wu tang* (modified), *Shen qi di huang tang* (modified) 参芪地黄汤(加味), *Qi shen yi qi di wan* 芪参益气滴丸, *Zhi dan jiang tang* capsule 丹蛭降糖胶囊, *Tong xin luo* capsule 通心络胶囊 and *Fu fang xue shuan tong* capsule 复方血栓通胶囊 may enhance the anti-albuminuric effect of ACEi/ARB. Moreover, *Shen qi di huang tang* (modified), *Fu fang xue shuan tong* capsule and *Dong chong xia cao* preparation reduced the SCr level when used with ACEi/ARB, and the effect of *Dong chong xia cao* preparation 冬虫夏草制剂 was only apparent when treatment durations exceeded three months.

Compared to ACEi/ARB, *Liu wei di huang wan* (modified) 六味地黄丸加减 in combination with ACEi/ARB did not produce additional benefits. When it was compared to ACEi/ARB, *Liu wei di huang wan* (modified) showed a greater effect on reducing albuminuria excretion.

The CHM treatments used in the included studies were unlikely to result in serious AEs, but may have been associated with gastro-intestinal upset and discomfort. Patients with DKD receiving CHM treatments who experienced vomiting and/or diarrhoea should be monitored for water and electrolyte disturbances. In addition, CHM appeared to reduce the incidence of dry couch caused by ACEi.

There are a number of limitations that should be noted. The original studies were at risk of selection and performance bias due to lack of blinding and insufficient reporting regarding randomisation and allocation. The meta-analysis largely focused on the overall effect of CHM on different outcomes, and CHM treatment details, such as formula ingredients, herb dosage and treatment duration, varied from study to study. Not surprisingly therefore, substantial heterogeneity was detected. Furthermore, all studies examined surrogate outcomes over relatively short time periods. The long-term effects of CHM on patient-level and patient-reported outcomes are unknown. Whether the short-term improvements in SCr concentration, albuminuria excretion and other surrogate outcomes observed with CHM in this meta-analysis would lead to long-term patient benefits remains uncertain.

References

1. Liu X, Liu L, Chen P, Zhou L, *et al.* (2014) Clinical trials of traditional Chinese medicine in the treatment of diabetic nephropathy-a systematic review based on a subgroup analysis. *J Ethnopharmacol* **151**(2): 810–819.
2. 冯新格, 曾艺鹏, 郭亚芳. (2013) 中西医结合治疗早期糖尿病肾病的荟萃分析. 河南中医 **33**(B10): 129–130.
3. 张颖. (2013) 中西医结合治疗早期糖尿病肾病的系统评价. 辽宁中医药大学. 学位论文.
4. 李绍钦. (2009) 中医络病理论与早期糖尿病肾病的相关研究. 广州中医药大学. 博士学位论文.
5. 谢豪杰, 严美花, 张乐, 肖雅, 赵晓山, 罗仁. (2011) 益气养阴活血法联合 ACEI 或 ARB 类药物治疗早期 2 型糖尿病肾病的系统评价. 中华中医药学刊 **29**(10): 2233–2236.
6. Higgins J, Green S. (eds.) (2011) *Cochrane Handbook for Systematic Reviews of Interventions Version 5.1.0* (The Cochrane Collaboration). Retrieved from http://www.cochrane-Handbook.org.

References for Included Chinese Herbal Medicine Clinical Studies

Study Number	References
H1	陈茜, 龚英. (2007) 益气养阴活血汤加灌肠治疗早期糖肾病疗效观察. 辽宁中医杂志 **34**(8): 1072–1073.
H2	颜秀芸. (2012) 清热利湿通络法治疗早期糖尿病肾病的临床研究. 南京中医药大学. 学位论文.
H3	高俊杰, 杨洪庆, 汪芳丽, 庞玲, 苏志国, 杨洪娟. (2013) 归芪升降散治疗 2 型糖尿病早期糖尿病肾病疗效观察. 河北中医药学报 **28**(3): 22–23.
H4	蒋文高, 洪兵. (2014) 芪参益气滴丸联合替米沙坦治疗糖尿病早期肾病的效果观察及对血清 SSA, IL-6 及 TNF-α 水平的影响. 中成药 **36**(9): 1822–1826.
H5	李宇丹, 丁志胜. (2009) 中西医结合治疗早期糖尿病肾病的近期疗效观察. 中国中西医结合肾病杂志 **10**(12): 1098–1099.
H6	申志祥, 孙世竹, 蒋娟娟, 刘燕, 高雪艳, 周丽萍, 陈燕. (2014) 中西药合用治疗早期糖尿病肾病 62 例临床观察. 江苏中医药 **46**(6): 43–44.
H7	严健如, 谢志芬. (2010) 中药联合卡托普利治疗早期糖尿病肾病的临床观察. 中医药导报 **16**(3): 29–30.
H8	雷秋娥. (2007) 中西医结合治疗早期糖尿病肾病 62 例的临床观察. 中外健康文摘·医药月刊 **4**(12): 218–219.
H9	刘国祥. (2014) 中医辩证结合氯沙坦方案治疗糖尿病肾病的疗效及对肾功能和血脂代谢的影响. 中国医药指南 **12**(23): 275–276.
H10	苏勇, 刘绛, 苏月南. (2012) 贝那普利合用益肾固精活血中药保护糖尿病肾病III期患者残存肾功能的临床研究. 国际医药卫生导报 **18**(9): 1248–1250.
H11	王凤丽, 陈志强, 王月华, 张江华, 李黎莉, 李林林, 张雪云. (2012) 益气养阴消癥通络方治疗早期糖尿病肾病临床观察. 中国中西医结合杂志 **32**(1): 35–37.
H12	项晓骏. (2010) 益气养阴活血法治疗糖尿病肾病的临床疗效分析. 中外医疗 **6**: 76.
H13	陈雪兰, 丘余良, 阮诗玮. (2011) 益肾降浊冲剂对脾肾气虚型糖尿病肾病III期患者尿微量白蛋白的影响. 中国中西医结合肾病杂志 **12**(12): 1066–1068.
H14	戴晓霞. (2001) 益气化瘀法治疗早期糖尿病肾病的临床观察. 中医药学报 **29**(2): 15.
H15	吕勇, 赵莉, 任克军. (2007) 雷氏丹参片对糖尿病肾病肾损害实验指标影响的临床研究. 中成药 **29**(3): 335–337.

(Continued)

(Continued)

Study Number	References
H16	马绍杰, 吕永恒, 陈冬, 王志文. (2004) 金芪降糖片对早期糖尿病肾病肾脏的保护作用. 四川中医 **9**: 39–40.
H17	王光明, 王志高. (2009) 益气养阴, 活血通络法治疗早期糖尿病肾病 63 例. 甘肃中医 **6**: 24–26.
H18	阳慧林. (2009) 尿毒清颗粒治疗早期糖尿病肾病的疗效观察. 右江医学 **37**(2): 142–143.
H19	杨嘉陵, 钱妍. (2015) 降糖保肾汤对早期糖尿病肾病干预的临床研究. 重庆医学 **44**(7): 973–975.
H20	赵红心, 孙文森. (2014) 当归补血汤加味治疗早期糖尿病肾病疗效研究. 河北中医药学报 **29**(2): 22–23.
H21	陈翠萍, 冯其斌. (2008) 蒙诺联合通心络胶囊治疗早期糖尿病肾病 31 例疗效观察. 新中医 **40**(5): 27–28.
H22	邱阜生, 杨燕, 杨茜, 贺玉珍. (2003) 糖肾清Ⅰ号治疗糖尿病肾病临床研究. 天津中医药 **20**(2): 21–22.
H23	高雪艳, 孙世竹, 刘燕, 周丽平, 蒋娟娟, 陈燕, 申志详. (2014) 肾糖康合剂联合西药治疗早期糖尿病肾病的临床研究. 实用老年医学 **28**(1): 43–45.
H24	何萍, 鲁冰冬. (2012) 缬沙坦联合金水宝胶囊治疗 2 型糖尿病肾病的疗效观察. 中国民康医学 **24**(12): 1452–1453.
H25	梁文俊. (2004) 降糖保肾合剂治疗早期糖尿病肾病临床研究. 北京中医药大学. 学位论文.
H26	梁永, 张研燕, 董杨颖, 邱振华, 黄金波. (2008) 益肾降糖汤治疗早期糖尿病肾病疗效观察. 中国中医急症 **17**(3): 312, 320.
H27	彭书渊, 黄廷荣. (2010) 中西医结合治疗早期糖尿病肾病的临床观察. 湖北中医杂志 **32**(7): 16–17.
H28	时红波. (2010) 培哚普利联合金水宝治疗早期 2 型糖尿病肾病临床观察. 中国实用医刊 **37**(7): 46–47.
H29	司圣海. (2012) 益气养阴活血法拟方联合西药治疗糖尿病肾病疗效观察. 中医药临床杂志 **24**(2): 121–122.
H30	王和强, 张太坤, 符莹, 廖信茜, 周湧, 邓淦林, 邓少奇. (2014) 中药糖通饮方对早期糖尿病肾病患者血清血管内皮生长因子的影响. 长春中医药大学学报 **30**(2): 298–300.
H31	王和强, 张太坤, 符莹, 廖信茜, 周湧, 邓淦林, 邓少奇. (2014) 中药糖通饮方治疗早期糖尿病肾病患者临床观察. 天津中医药大学学报 **33**(5): 267–269.

(Continued)

(Continued)

Study Number	References
H32	武慧, 杜宏武, 谢道俊. (2001) 益气养阴活血通腑法为主治疗老年早期糖尿病肾病 31 例. 安徽中医学院学报 **20**(1): 16–18.
H33	夏晶, 高彦彬, 张涛静. (2010) 益气养阴, 化痰逐瘀法治疗早期糖尿病肾病 20 例临床研究. 安徽中医学院学报 **29**(2): 22–25.
H34	肖振忠, 孙宏君. (2010) 黄葵胶囊联合缬沙坦对早期糖尿病肾病患者微量白蛋白尿的影响. 现代中西医结合杂志 **19**(3): 263–264.
H35	徐德颐, 徐珏, 凌青. (2005) 保肾汤治疗 2 型糖尿病早期肾病临床观察. 吉林中医药 **25**(8): 12–13.
H36	俞荣强. (2006) 福辛普利联合冬虫夏草制剂对早期 2 型糖尿病肾病微量白蛋白尿的影响. 中华医学实践杂志 **5**(5): 493–494.
H37	曾尚校, 张丽梅. (2010) 厄贝沙坦联合金水宝胶囊治疗老年 2 型糖尿病肾病的临床疗效观察. 中国医师进修杂志 **33**(24): 35–37.
H38	张又云, 黄河清. (2002) 抵当汤改良方治疗早期糖尿病肾病的研究. 现代中西医结合杂志 **11**(21): 2091–2092.
H39	翟晓丽, 许筠, 苏建平, 张星, 程保智, 谢华. (2008) 芪龙益肾汤对早期糖尿病肾病治疗作用的临床观察. 中华中医药学会第二十一届全国中医肾病学术会议: 241–243.
H40	周晖, 商学征, 谢培凤, 关崧, 盛彤, 易文明, 张涛静, 高彦彬. (2009) 益气养阴解毒通络法治疗早期糖尿病肾病的临床研究. 天津中医药. **26**(2): 100–102.
H41	高彦彬, 赵慧珍, 关崧, 周晖, 庚及娣, 谢培凤, 赵翠芳, 商学征, 郝青春. (2006) 糖肾宁治疗气阴两虚, 络脉瘀滞型早期糖尿病肾病临床研究. 中华中医药杂志 **21**(7): 409–411.
H42	黄海泉. (2000) 百令胶囊治疗 II 型糖尿病伴微白蛋白尿的临床观察. 临床交流 **9**(8): 43.
H43	夏成云, 周京国, 谢建平, 康后生, 张国元, 刘福. (2004) 茶色素对早期糖尿病肾病患者血尿转化生长因子 β1 的影响. 中国中西医结合急救杂志 **11**(5): 297–300.
H44	李琳. (2006) 补阳还五汤加减治疗早期糖尿病肾病 34 例临床观察. 中医药导报 **12**(6): 16–18.
H45	叶赏和, 陈跃华, 傅晓骏, 刘瑾, 郎旭军, 李旭升. (2006) 银杏叶提取物治疗早期糖尿病肾病的临床观察. 中国医院药学杂志 **26**(9): 1182–1183.
H46	张永, 张建鄂, 吴平勇, 张庆红. (2007) 绞股蓝总甙与缬沙坦治疗早期糖尿病肾病的对比研究. 郧阳医学院学报 **26**(4): 199–202.

(Continued)

(*Continued*)

Study Number	References
H47	饶祖华, 余颖, 李小青, 庞晓红, 任跃忠. (2008) 芪蛭降糖胶囊治疗早期糖尿病肾病 34 例临床观察. 浙江临床医学 **10**(7): 909–910.
H48	郭聂涛, 刘琳娜, 顾向明, 朱小华, 杜国有, 杨进. (2009) 益气养阴活血方对早期糖尿病肾病患者胱抑素 c 水平的影响. 实用中西医结合临床 **9**(6): 12–14.
H49	Li Xusheng, Zheng Weiying, Lou Shixian, Lu Xiaowen, Ye Shanghe (李旭升, 郑伟英, 楼时先, 陆小文, 叶赏和). (2009) Effect of Ginkgo Leaf Extract on Vascular Endothelial Function in Patients with Early Stage Diabetic Nephropathy. *Chin J Integr Med* **15**(1): 26–29.
H50	林道强, 陈文. (2009) 中西医结合治疗早期糖尿病肾病 66 例. 南京中医药大学学报 **25**(5): 394–395.
H51	杨帅, 刘湘红. (2009) 黄葵胶囊配合西药治疗早期糖尿病肾病 32 例临床观察. 河北中医 **31**(4): 600–602.
H52	蔡景英, 王艳芬, 曹萍. (2010) 尿毒清颗粒治疗早期糖尿病肾病临床研究. 实用糖尿病杂志 **6**(4): 37–38.
H53	丛艳. (2011) 复方滋肾饮治疗早期糖尿病肾病 25 例. 中国中医药现代远程教育 **9**(19): 153–154.
H54	崔冰, 马继伟. (2011) 六味地黄丸方治疗早期糖尿病肾病 33 例. 中国中医急症 **20**(5): 804.
H55	佟丽娟. (2011) 益气养阴活血汤治疗早期糖尿病肾病 40 例. 实用中医内科杂志 **25**(6): 85–86.
H56	肖雪云, 周茹, 陈发盛. (2011) 尿毒清颗粒治疗早期糖尿病肾病 40 例疗效观察. 新中医 **43**(8): 48–49.
H57	陈思洁, 龚保文, 黄润山, 王丹阳, 蔡凯鹏. (2012) 温阳化饮方治疗早期糖尿病肾病并胸腔积液疗效观察. 实用医学杂志 **28**(9): 1542–1544.
H58	康广水. (2012) 自拟芪蛭地黄汤治疗早期糖尿病肾病疗效观察. 中国中医药现代远程教育 **10**(7): 121.
H59	沈琼, 王飞. (2012) 血脂康治疗早期糖尿病肾病疗效观察. 实用糖尿病杂志 **8**(2): 15–16.
H60	宋林宏, 张德宪, 龚敏, 孙守芳, 赵英英, 陈文文. (2012) 滋阴泄浊方治疗糖尿病肾病临床观察. 辽宁中医药大学学报 **14**(6): 170–171.
H61	曾翠青. (2012) 益气活血法治疗早期糖尿病肾病的疗效观察. 现代预防医学 **39**(18): 4881–4882, 4884.
H62	邓顺有, 范翠, 张征, 陈小燕, 谭愈昱. (2013) 滋肾活血法联合厄贝沙坦治疗早期糖尿病肾病的临床疗效. 中国老年学杂志 **33**(1): 37–39.

(*Continued*)

(*Continued*)

Study Number	References
H63	焦颖华, 邢磊, 田发明, 崔立华, 王志文, 孙尧, 李向男. (2013)解聚复肾宁治疗早期 2 型糖尿病肾病. 中国实验方剂学杂志 **19**(23): 317–320.
H64	吴敏, 张文萍, 朱成晟, 王晶晶, 傅玲玲. (2013) 滋肾清利通络法配合治疗早期糖尿病肾病 26 例临床观察. 江苏中医药 **45**(6): 27–28.
H65	金俊涛. (2014) 益气化瘀汤治疗早期糖尿病肾病临床效果观察. 亚太传统医药 **10**(8): 122–123.
H66	马婕. (2014) 益气养阴清热活血法治疗早期糖尿病肾病的疗效及对血液流变学的影响. 吉林中医药 **34**(12): 1225–1228.
H67	汪何. (2014) 益气升清方治疗早期糖尿病肾病的临床观察. 湖北中医杂志 **36**(5): 5–6.
H68	张生计, 陈静. (2014) 柴苓汤治疗早期糖尿病肾病临床分析. 内蒙古中医药: 32.
H69	张震宇, 李耀威, 苗润. (2014) 坎地沙坦酯片联合金水宝治疗 2 型糖尿病早期肾病疗效观察. 广东药学院学报 **30**(2): 241–244.
H70	郭蔚, 但刚, 陈钰, 薛萍, 卢蓉. (2009) 肾炎康复片与坎地沙坦酯治疗糖尿病肾病的对照研究. 西南国防医药 **19**(7): 681–683.
H71	王建华, 邵雪珍, 熊玮, 肖凤英, 伊磊亚, 付德辉. (2013) 早期糖尿病肾病中西医干预的临床疗效比较. 湖北中医杂志 **35**(6): 13–14.
H72	鲍红娟. (2011) 中药联用厄贝沙坦治疗糖尿病肾病微量白蛋白尿期的疗效观察. 中华中医药学刊 **29**(3): 540–542.
H73	鲍正宏, 朱江涛, 鲍惠君, 刘海芳. (2008) 糖肾 2 号方与依那普利联用治疗早期糖尿病肾病的临床对照观察. 北京中医药大学学报 **15**(6): 22–23.
H74	曹瑞. (2010) 益气养阴活血中药治疗早期糖尿病肾病 60 例临床观察. 安徽医药 **14**(10): 1211–1212.
H75	曹小川. (2015) 缬沙坦联合百令胶囊治疗早期糖尿病肾病的效果分析. 中国当代医药 **22**(4): 97–98, 101.
H76	陈广, 屠青年, 李伶俐, 黄召谊, 董慧. (2014) 三七交泰丸联合洛丁新片治疗糖尿病肾病30例临床观察. 中医杂志 **55**(20): 1735–1738.
H77	陈军. (2001) 中西医结合治疗早期糖尿病肾病临床观察. 湖北中医杂志 **23**(11): 21.
H78	陈静媛. (2006) 中西医结合治疗早期糖尿病肾病的临床观察. 实用糖尿病杂志 **2**(2): 36–37.
H79	陈敏. (2008) 中西医结合治疗老年早期糖尿病肾病的临床观察. 第六次全国中西医结合中青年学术研讨会: 321–324.

(*Continued*)

(**Continued**)

Study Number	References
H80	陈伟锦. (2011) 至灵胶囊联合厄贝沙坦治疗早期糖尿病肾病的疗效观察. 现代医院 **11**(8): 57–58.
H81	陈文文. (2010) 糖肾平治疗糖尿病肾病（III期）的临床研究. 山东中医药大学. 学位论文.
H82	翟晓丽, 许筠, 韩业宏, 苏建平, 程保智, 谢华, 张茹. (2013) 益气养阴化瘀中药对糖尿病肾病患者血清 no, et-1 水平的影响. 中国中西医结合肾病杂志 **14**(10): 872–874.
H83	丁涛. (2014) 厄贝沙坦与金水宝对糖尿病肾病的临床疗效观察. 数理医药学杂志 **27**(2): 207–208.
H84	窦晓丽, 武金强, 韩丽丽, 于似月, 扈瑞春. (2012) 自拟益气活血方治疗糖尿病肾病的临床研究. 山西医药杂志·上半月 **41**(5): 440–442.
H85	杜守作. (2011) 厄贝沙坦联合丹参治疗早期糖尿病肾病的临床观察. 海南医学 **19**: 17–18.
H86	法文喜. (2014) 加味桂枝茯苓丸治疗糖尿病肾病的临床观察. 特别健康: 下 **7**: 525–526.
H87	范艳艳. (2012) 芪药糖肾消治疗早期糖尿病肾病的临床研究. 南京中医药大学. 学位论文.
H88	冯琼邵, 邵跃斌, 冉建民, 杨秀文, 劳干诚. (2008) 补阳还五汤联合替米沙坦治疗早期糖尿病肾病疗效观察. 广东医学 **29**(8): 1414–1415.
H89	高娅丽. (2013) "通脉降脂丸" 对糖尿病肾病早期气虚血瘀型的疗效观察. 云南中医学院. 学位论文.
H90	龚翠芬, 乔小利, 魏金花, 胡宝峰. (2009) 当归补血汤加味配合贝那普利治疗早期糖尿病肾病 60 例. 陕西中医 **30**(8): 974–976.
H91	韩晶晶, 陈霞波, 龚文波, 唐亚军. (2015) 参芪地黄汤联合缬沙坦治疗早期气阴两虚型糖尿病肾病的临床疗效观察. 中华中医药学刊 **33**(4): 986–990.
H92	洪小平. (2011) 益气敛微汤联用贝那普利治疗早期糖尿病肾病的临床研究. 中国中医药科技 **18**(2): 91–92.
H93	黄赐平. (2014) 金水宝胶囊合复方丹参滴丸治疗老年早期糖尿病肾病 48 例. 光明中医 **29**(6): 1304–1305.
H94	黄积仓, 张玉峰, 王晓瑜, 武俊斌, 王丽, 毛玉娟. (2010) 虫草菌粉联合银杏叶片对糖尿病肾病III期患者蛋白尿的影响. 中医药学报 **38**(1): 57–59.
H95	贾振武. (2014) 地黄叶总苷胶囊联合氯沙坦钾片治疗早期糖尿病肾病的疗效观察. 中国医药指南 **12**(12): 263–264.

(*Continued*)

(*Continued*)

Study Number	References
H96	江岸林, 曹爱萍, 褚小燕, 朱铭卿, 张永建. (2010) 发酵虫草菌粉 (CS-4) 联合厄贝沙坦治疗早期 2 型糖尿病肾病临床观察. 中国中西医结合肾病杂志 **11**(11): 994–995.
H97	金鸥阳, 高磊平. (2013) 摄精消白胶囊配合治疗糖尿病肾病 30 例临床研究. 江苏中医药 **45**(4): 33–34.
H98	琚枫, 黄亚莲, 符茂雄. (2013) 中药联合洛汀新治疗糖尿病肾病微量白蛋白尿 25 例. 江西中医药 **44**(7): 39–41.
H99	孔垂红. (2014) 通络解毒方联合雷公藤多苷治疗早期糖尿病肾病疗效观察. 新中医 **46**(7): 147–149.
H100	雷水红, 李经, 赖晓阳, 张美英, 张笠, 熊燕. (2009) 安博维联合金水宝治疗非高血压糖尿病肾病疗效观察. 山东医药 **49**(1): 98–99.
H101	李红萍. (2012) 厄贝沙坦联合消解通络固肾汤治疗糖尿病肾病临床观察. 现代中西医结合杂志 **21**(21): 2338–2339.
H102	黎晶晶. (2013) 健脾益肾, 清热利湿活血法治疗早期糖尿病肾病的临床疗效研究. 南京中医药大学. 学位论文.
H103	李六生, 刘建社, 陈建娜, 胡生琼. (2006) 缬沙坦联合大黄治疗糖尿病肾病的疗效. 实用医学杂志 **13**: 1580–1582.
H104	李青, 韩宇博. (2014) 金匮肾气丸联合美卡素治疗III期糖尿病肾病的临床研究. 光明中医 **29**(3): 576–578.
H105	李晓莉. (2010) 科素亚联合百令胶囊治疗早期糖尿病肾病的疗效观察. 中国中医药咨讯 **2**(30): 184–185.
H106	李永国, 戴国军. (2014) 中西医结合治疗早期糖尿病肾病疗效观察. 现代中西医结合杂志 **2**(16): 1776–1777.
H107	李勇坚. (2009) 补中益气汤加味合厄贝沙坦对早期糖尿病肾病的干预治疗临床研究. 云南中医药杂志 **30**(7): 10–12.
H108	李奕升, 郭洪波, 罗辉娥, 马厚蓉. (2014) 健脾祛湿法治疗早期糖尿病肾病的临床研究. 山东中医杂志 **33**(11): 891–893.
H109	李月婷. (2014) 黄葵胶囊联合缬沙坦治疗糖尿病肾病临床效果分析. 社区医学杂志 **12**(15): 36–37.
H110	李业展. (2010) 中西医结合治疗早期糖尿病肾病 34 例临床观察. 江苏中医药 **42**(6): 33–34.
H111	赵明, 梁淼, 肖宏. (2008) 氯沙坦联合红景天治疗早期糖尿病肾病的临床研究. 中国实用内科杂志 **8**(5): 230–232.
H112	刘翠萍, 李敏娟. (2011) 厄贝沙坦联合百令胶囊治疗早期糖尿病肾病的疗效观察. 河北医药 **33**(11): 1661–1662.

(*Continued*)

(Continued)

Study Number	References
H113	刘承琴, 赵建群. (2003) 滋肾健脾化瘀方治疗早期糖尿病肾病 41 例. 山东中医杂志 (**11**): 648–649.
H114	刘明伟. (2011) 氯沙坦联合百灵胶囊治疗糖尿病肾病的疗效评价. 中国误诊学杂志 **11**(26): 6336.
H115	刘志伟, 张丽华, 陈沛林. (2009) 中西医结合治疗早期糖尿病肾病 40 例临床观察. 江苏中医药 **41**(3): 37–38.
H116	陆标明, 陈汉礼. (2009) 滋肾降糖饮加瑞格列奈治疗早期糖尿病肾病疗效观察. 实用中医药杂志 **25**(7): 459–460.
H117	卢远征. (2009) 活血化瘀法治疗早期糖尿病肾病的临床疗效观察. 广州中医药大学. 学位论文.
H118	罗方, 胡江平. (2011) 百令胶囊辅助治疗早期糖尿病肾病临床观察. 药物流行病学杂志 **20**(7): 334–336.
H119	罗方, 曹珊, 孙新宇. (2011) 百令胶囊联合厄贝沙坦治疗早期糖尿病肾病的临床研究. 中医学报 **26**(4): 466–467.
H120	吕泳城. (2011) 血府逐瘀汤对2型糖尿病肾病III期患者 CRP 及尿 CTGFf 影响的临床研究. 福建中医药大学. 学位论文.
H121	马晓莉. (2014) 西红康方治疗糖尿病肾病III期气阴两虚兼血瘀型的临床研究. 新疆医科大学. 学位论文.
H122	毛春谱, 李小毅, 张红梅, 林桂芬. (2009) 银杏叶提取物治疗早期糖尿病肾病的临床研究. 中国综合临床 **25**(3): 299–301.
H123	梅莎莎, 宋恩峰, 项琼. (2014) 糖脂同调治疗早期糖尿病肾病临床观察. 辽宁中医药大学学报 **16**(9): 93–95.
H124	彭仙珍, 沈三英, 宋小红, 肖政, 李文华. (2007) 缬沙坦联合通心络胶囊治疗糖尿病肾病的临床疗效分析. 医药导报 **26**(3): 268–269.
H125	钱力维, 杨升杰, 陈瑜瑜. (2012) 肾炎舒胶囊联合厄贝沙坦治疗早期糖尿病肾病 35 例. 安徽中医学院学报 **31**(3): 29–31.
H126	裘磊, 郑军状, 郑建芳, 陆新烈. (2013) 健脾益气活血方结合常规疗法治疗糖尿病肾病疗效观察. 上海中医药杂志 **47**(3): 42–43.
H127	师魏霞. (2009) 补肾活血汤治疗糖尿病肾病的临床观察. 中华中医药杂志 **24**(8): 1102–1103.
H128	宋玉山. (2007) 健脾补肾活血法治疗早期糖尿病肾病临床研究. 河北医科大学. 学位论文.
H129	田虎. (2014) 温阳益气养阴活血方治疗早期糖尿病肾病的疗效观察. 黑龙江中医药 **5**: 27–28.

(Continued)

(Continued)

Study Number	References
H130	仝用, 冀玲琴, 李艳颖, 姚琼, 杨西强, 曹阿丹. (2012) 雷公藤多苷治疗糖尿病肾病III期疗效分析. 中国医药 **7**(11): 1418–1420.
H131	汪朝振, 张太阳. (2013) 固肾温阳法联合厄贝沙坦治疗早期糖尿病肾病的临床观察. 实用中西医结合临床 **13**(1): 19–20.
H132	王海燕, 王小强, 周东海, 邵桂军, 杨靖. (2009) 复元保肾汤治疗早期糖尿病肾病 48 例临床观察. 河北中医 **31**(6): 838–839.
H133	王玲琳, 沈世豪, 应培珍, 王孝妹, 周青. (2007) 氯沙坦联合通心络对 2 型糖尿病患者肾功能的影响. 疑难病杂志 **6**(2): 85–87.
H134	王妮娜, 曾晓聪. (2012) 复方血栓通胶囊与氯沙坦钾联合治疗早期糖尿病肾病的疗效观察. 临床和实验医学杂志 **11**(12): 928–929, 931.
H135	王文豪. (2013) 温脏扶正祛邪方治疗早期糖尿病肾病的临床观察. 广州中医药大学. 学位论文.
H136	王玉英. (2008) 自拟保肾汤与洛汀新治疗早期糖尿病肾病的临床观察. 中华中医药学刊 **26**(6): 1354–1356.
H137	韦劲, 方朝晖, 彭代银, 陈勇, 祝峻峰, 高晓坤. (2010) 复方丹皮煎剂治疗气阴两虚型早期糖尿病肾病的临床研究. 中国药房 **21**(3): 255–257.
H138	吴琼, 杨柏新. (2010) 褐藻多糖硫酸酯与贝那普利联合应用治疗早期糖尿病肾病. 临床军医杂志 **38**(5): 743–745.
H139	吴卫东. (2011) 中西医结合治疗早期糖尿病肾病59例临床研究. 中国中医药咨讯 **3**(23): 309.
H140	谢辉, 朱琳, 黄霖, 肖洁, 肖云, 刘汉欣. (2011) 降糖保肾方联合厄贝沙坦治疗早期糖尿病肾病的临床研究. 中国中西医结合肾病杂志 **12**(7): 616–619.
H141	谢秀仪. (2014) 降糖三黄片治疗糖尿病肾病早期临床疗效观察. 广州中医药大学. 学位论文.
H142	辛传伟, 黄萍, 田云龙, 郑柳娟. (2014) 消渴平合剂对早期糖尿病肾病患者 VEGF 的影响作用研究. 中华中医药学刊 **32**(3): 559–561.
H143	徐会彬, 周刚鑫, 赵英红, 刘慧君, 姚春杰. (2007) 中西医结合治疗早期糖尿病肾病的研究. 现代中西医结合杂志 **16**(21): 2965–2966, 2968.
H144	徐小琳, 薛少清, 陈仁富, 徐冠雄. (2014) 氯沙坦联合百令胶囊黄芪颗粒治疗早期糖尿病肾病的疗效观察. 中外医疗**5**: 30–31.
H145	杨春华. (2013) 金水宝胶囊联合氯沙坦治疗早期糖尿病肾病疗效观察. 现代中西医结合杂志**1**: 65–66.

(Continued)

(*Continued*)

Study Number	References
H146	杨坷. (2012) 加味芪黄饮对糖尿病肾病 acr 影响的研究. 广州中医药大学. 学位论文.
H147	姚定国, 魏佳平. (2003) 桃红二子汤合一平苏治疗早期糖尿病肾病. 浙江中西医结合杂志 **13**(8): 474–476.
H148	姚军, 刘俊峰. (2015) 黄芪精口服液联合卡托普利治疗早期糖尿病肾病的临床观察. 中国医药指南 **13**(3): 219–220.
H149	叶健波, 刘志梅, 李剑军, 林华征, 陆军. (2012) 百令胶囊联合坎地沙坦酯治疗早期糖尿病肾病的临床观察. Internal Medicine China **7**(6): 612–613.
H150	玉山江·艾克木, 哈丽达·木沙. (2015) 西红康对糖尿病肾病III期患者同型半胱氨酸水平的影响. 中国中医基础医学杂志 **21**(2): 189–191, 222.
H151	袁飞, 刘国辉, 林宏初. (2008) 中西医结合治疗早期糖尿病肾病的临床研究. 中国保健营养·临床医学学刊 **17**(22): 13–15.
H152	张灵建, 洪波. (2014) 九味糖肾汤对糖尿病肾病患者血郁胶原, 层粘连蛋白表达的影响. 浙江中西医结合杂志 **24**(3): 211–213.
H153	张书申, 王芳, 乔苏民. (2007) 脑心通胶囊联合福辛普利治疗早期糖尿病肾病. 中西医结合心脑血管病杂志 **5**(12): 1180–1181.
H154	张彤, 盖云, 杨晓萍. (2011) 中西医结合治疗早期糖尿病肾病 30 例临床研究. 江苏中医药 **43**(7): 27–28.
H155	张新利, 吕芹, 吴瑞格. (2011) 复方丹参滴丸联合科素亚治疗早期老年 2 型糖尿病肾病疗效观察. 中国误诊学杂志 **11**(12): 2798.
H156	张玉峰, 黄机仓, 杨国栋, 武俊斌, 王丽, 毛玉娟, 景俊, 雷明春. (2012) 生脉散合归脾汤加减治疗糖尿病肾病III期气阴两虚型 48 例临床观察. 甘肃中医学院学报 **29**(6): 33–35.
H157	郑文静. (2012) 中西医结合治疗糖尿病肾病临床观察. 山西中医 **28**(10): 32–33.
H158	周忠海, 王卫松, 高俊杰, 李丽华. (2012) "益气活血通络汤"治疗早期糖尿病肾病 57 例临床研究. 江苏中医药 **44**(4): 18–19.
H159	朱娜, 蔡颖娴, 房春花, 曹雪明, 吴玉, 汪彬彬. (2012) 温肾解毒祛瘀方对早期糖尿病肾病患者血浆内皮素和 p-选择素的影响. 现代中西医结合杂志 **21**(11): 1146–1147.
H160	张洪勤. (2012) 脾肾双补法治疗糖尿病肾病 38 例临床观察. 中医药导报 **18**(2): 38–40.

(*Continued*)

(Continued)

Study Number	References
H161	陈宇斌. (2015) 益气通淋胶囊联合氯沙坦治疗早期糖尿病肾病效果观察. 白求恩医学杂志 **13**(1): 103–104.
H162	董津含. (2013) 益肾康颗粒治疗早餐糖尿病肾病 60 例安全性研究. 辽宁中医药大学. 学位论文.
H163	郭兆安, 于春江, 李悦, 姜蓓蓓, 彭书玲. (2013) 芪蛭降糖胶囊治疗糖尿病肾病III期的临床研究. 中国中西医结合急救杂志 **20**(5): 261–265.
H164	彭继升. (2007) 芪卫颗粒治疗早期糖尿病肾病的临床研究. 北京中医药大学. 学位论文.
H165	施进宝, 黄宝英, 郑瑞平, 刘芳, 蔡奕奇. (2014) 参芪丹糖肾消方治疗气阴两虚夹瘀型早期糖尿病肾病 40 例. 福建中医药 **45**(4): 13–17.
H166	徐蓉娟, 唐红, 朱良争, 钟家宝, 胡健炜, 李红, 杨华. (1999) 治糖保肾冲剂治疗糖尿病早期肾病 32 例临床观察. 中国中西医结合杂志 **19**(10): 624–625.
H167	曾雪榕. (2008) 芪药地黄汤治疗糖尿病肾病III期（气阴两虚型）的临床疗效观察. 福建中医学院. 学位论文.
H168	张志忠, 王彩霞, 魏建红, 徐升. (2009) 益气养阴合剂治疗糖尿病肾病临床研究. 中华中医药学刊 **27**(8): 1755–1757.
H169	周广举. (2013) 渴络欣联合厄贝沙坦治疗早期糖尿病肾病蛋白尿的临床研究. 临床合理用药杂志 **6**(12A): 20–21.
H170	朱丹平. (2005) 中西医结合治疗糖尿病肾病3期的临床研究. 成都中医药大学. 学位论文.
H171	朱秀. (2011) 益气养阴活血方治疗糖尿病肾病 30 例疗效观察. 中国医药指南 **9**(20): 147–149.
H172	魏娜, 常万松, 薛迪中, 沈学飞. (2012) 血脂康对早期糖尿病肾病患者氧化应激的影响. 中国全科医学 **15**(6C): 2085–2087.
H173	杨力, 檀增衡, 李玉坤. (2014) 芪明颗粒配合常规疗法治疗早期糖尿病肾病 71 例临床观察. 中医药导报 **20**(6): 52–53.
H174	范译文. (2010) 芪葵颗粒干预早期 2 型糖尿病肾病的临床研究. 南京中医药大学. 学位论文.
H175	谢绍锋, 黄莉吉, 刘敬顺, 余江毅, 王小超. (2011) 长期应用养阴和络中药对早期糖尿病肾病患者尿微量白蛋白肌酐比值的影响. 江苏中医药 **43**(9): 19–20.
H176	高菁, 李靖, 莫世安, 庄杰, 来于. (2013) 益气养阴, 活血化瘀散结法治疗 2 型糖尿病肾病III, iv期气阴两虚夹瘀型 40 例临床研究. 世界中医药 **8**(5): 530–534

(Continued)

(*Continued*)

Study Number	References
H177	郭芳, 蓝元隆, 洪杨华. (2011) 益气养阴活血方治疗早期糖尿病肾病疗效观察. 福建中医药 **42**(6): 15–17.
H178	金叶, 万浩鹏, 张雨. (2012) 白术地黄汤治疗早期糖尿病肾病 38 例. 现代中西医结合杂志 **21**(29): 3239–3240.
H179	孔祥明, 梁炜. (2002) 大黄糖肾胶囊对早期糖尿病肾病的临床疗效. 现代医学 **30**(6): 363–365.
H180	李颖, 范晨, 王海英, 宋含平. (2011) 补阳还五汤对早期糖尿病肾病转化生长因子 β1(TGF-β1) 的作用. 中国医药导刊 **13**(4): 656–657.
H181	刘玲. (2005) 益气活血法对早期糖尿病肾病的干预研究. 南京中医药大学. 学位论文.
H182	刘孝琴, 李悦, 李雅楠. (2013) 益肾化湿颗粒对早期糖尿病肾病患者 CRP 及 IL-8 的影响. 中国中西医结合肾病杂志 **14**(6): 538–539.
H183	刘珍, 刘绛, 张绪生. (2007) 复方固肾冲剂治疗老年糖尿病肾病肾虚血瘀型蛋白尿 20 例总结. 湖南中医杂志 **23**(3): 23–25.
H184	吕秀群, 刘得华. (2012) 复方田参胶囊治疗早期糖尿病肾病疗效观察. 中医药临床杂志 **24**(12): 1195–1196.
H185	马丽. (2012) 金洪元学术思想与临床经验总结及糖肾通络方治疗糖尿病肾病的临床研究. 北京中医药大学. 学位论文.
H186	牛西武, 张兰, 侯宝华, 霍岩, 梁健. (2007) 益肾康对早期糖尿病肾病影响的临床研究. 实用中医内科杂志 **21**(1): 64–65.
H187	舒占钧, 王魁亮. (2007) 保元活血泄浊法治疗早期糖尿病肾病的临床研究. 新疆中医药 **25**(5): 11–15.
H188	宋艳丽, 李宗文, 王秋平. (2011) 益气养阴活血散结法治疗早期糖尿病肾病 30 例疗效观察. 医学信息·中旬刊**6**: 2833.
H189	王树亮, 刘清波. (2010) 健脾化瘀汤治疗早期糖尿病肾病的疗效分析. 中国中医药咨讯 **2**(32): 54.
H190	王玥. (2010) 益肾化瘀汤治疗早期糖尿病肾病临床观察. 新中医 **42**(12): 13–14.
H191	王玉红, 郭浩生. (2011) 益气养阴化瘀汤治疗早期糖尿病肾病 30 例疗效观察. 河北中医 **33**(8): 1132–1133.
H192	徐晓琴, 张效科, 薛金志, 刘国领. (2012) 益肾活血汤治疗糖尿病肾病早期 30 例总结. 湖南中医杂志 **28**(5): 38–39.
H193	叶芳. (2007) 糖肾安汤治疗早期糖尿病肾病临床观察. 国际中医中药杂志 **29**(4): 248–249.

(Continued)

(Continued)

Study Number	References
H194	袁放, 江缨, 郑和昕, 吴天凤, 陈业欢, 叶雄伟, 许雅萍. (2011) 自拟玉米须汤对早期糖尿病肾病的保护作用. 中华中医药学刊 **29**(11): 2468–2469.
H195	周鑫, 陈晓霞. (2010) 复方健胰颗粒治疗早期糖尿病肾病 50 例临床观察. 中医药临床杂志 **2**: 142–143.
H196	曹柏龙, 孙光荣. (2014) 运用孙光荣"三联药对"组方学术思想治疗早期糖尿病肾病的临床观察. 北京中医药 **33**(1): 10–12.
H197	邓远平, 吴义萍, 张绿平, 李梅, 卿永洪. (2013) 补肾活血化浊方治疗糖尿病肾病 30 例临床观察. 四川中医 **31**(10): 93–94.
H198	高天舒, 于世家, 李敬林. (1999) 中药早肾康治疗糖尿病肾病微量白蛋白尿 38 例. 辽宁中医学院学报 **1**(4): 41–42.
H199	郭建立, 张红伟. (2009) 糖肾饮治疗早期糖尿病肾病 26 例. 河南中医 **29**(5): 472–473.
H200	郭业新, 吕冬梅, 曹圣华, 王俊丽. (2007) 银杏叶提取物联合格列齐特, 二甲双胍治疗早期糖尿病肾病 32 例. 中国中西医结合肾病杂志 **8**(10): 607–608.
H201	靳瑞英. (2013) 滋阴通脉饮治疗早期糖尿病肾病临床观察. 实用中西医结合临床 **13**(7): 14–15.
H202	李建生. (1998) 大黄蟅虫丸对老年糖尿病早期肾病 TXB2 和 6-Keto-PGF_(1α) 的影响. 辽宁中医杂志 **25**(10): 465–467.
H203	刘保胜, 管淑琴, 逯继伟. (2014) 益气活血中药治疗糖尿病肾病 25 例. 中国药业 **23**(14): 99–100.
H204	刘孝琴, 王云枫, 李雅楠. (2013) 参芪地黄汤加味配合门冬胰岛素对早期 2 型糖尿病肾病负氮平衡的影响. 环球中医药 **6**(5): 366–368.
H205	刘艳峰, 郑朝霞, 胡天晓. (2014) 慢肾宁合剂治疗早期糖尿病肾病的疗效观察. 临床荟萃 **29**(7): 814–815.
H206	刘志伟, 安淑华, 叶春芳, 张丽华, 田丽, 马正云, 唐艳玲. (2013) 疏肝理气方治疗早期糖尿病肾病患者及对血管内皮功能的影响. 陕西中医 **33**(12): 1603–1605.
H207	马燕, 陈劲松, 张柏林. (2012) 益肾化瘀冲剂治疗早期糖尿病肾病临床观察及对 HCY 和 NAG 的影响. 天津中医药 **29**(4): 335–337.
H208	倪青, 张效科. (2009) 芪药消渴胶囊治疗早期糖尿病肾病 64 例临床观察. 北京中医药大学学报·中医临床版 **16**(4): 33–35.
H209	孙世宁, 黄红芳. (2004) 通心络胶囊对早期糖尿病肾病患者血浆, 尿内皮素的影响. 新中医 **36**(4): 32–33.

(Continued)

(*Continued*)

Study Number	References
H210	王小超, 刘克冕, 狄红杰, 冯栋年. (2009) 活血化瘀重剂治疗早期糖尿病肾病的疗效与机制探讨. 光明中医 **24**(11): 2060–2062.
H211	王秀芬, 赵苍朵, 顾连方, 李英. (2005) 加减补阳还五汤对早期糖尿病肾病的临床疗效及作用机制探讨. 中国中西医结合肾病杂志 **6**(5): 280–281.
H212	王秀芬, 赵苍朵, 张慧玲. (2006) 益气活血汤治疗早期糖尿病肾病 40 例疗效观察. 新中医 **38**(4): 46–47.
H213	魏金花. (2009) 益气逐瘀汤治疗早期糖尿病肾病的疗效观察. 亚太传统医药 **5**(10): 98–99.
H214	魏玲玲. (2004) 益气活血法治疗早期糖尿病肾病 30 例临床观察. 中医杂志 **45**(1): 39–40.
H215	肖丽红. (2009) 血脂康治疗早期糖尿病肾病疗效分析. 中国误诊学杂志 **9**(7): 1562.
H216	薛丽辉. (2002) 益气养阴活血法治疗早期糖尿病肾病探析. 辽宁中医杂志 **29**(3): 154.
H217	闫顺新, 郭小舟, 张玉军, 王金玲. (2015) 补肾固精方治疗阴阳两虚型早期糖尿病肾病临床研究. 中国中医药信息杂志**1**: 33–35.
H218	姚勇利. (2006) 乐脉颗粒对早期糖尿病肾病患者尿微量白蛋白排泄率的影响. 华西药学杂志 **21**(3): 310–311.
H219	于春军, 王祥生. (2010) 黄葵胶囊治疗早期糖尿病肾病的疗效观察. 中国中医急症 **19**(10): 1685–1709.
H220	张黎群, 李顺民, 董彦敏, 黄华. (2011) 活血降糖饮对糖尿病肾病患者尿微量白蛋白的影响. 中医学报 **26**(6): 715–717.
H221	张孙伟, 刘湘华. (2014) 活血补肾方联合西药治疗糖尿病肾病随机平行对照研究. 实用中医内科杂志 **28**(7): 129–131.
H222	张奕, 刘海霞, 程丽霞, 李红艳, 孟祥凤. (2009) 糖脉康治疗早期糖尿病肾病的临床观察. 亚太传统医药 **5**(9): 141–142.
H223	郑士荣, 张景红, 朱宇清, 蔡淦. (2002) 地灵丹对糖尿病肾病尿微量白蛋白排泄率及内皮素的影响. 深圳中西医结合杂志 **12**(5): 283–284.
H224	郑士荣, 张景红, 朱宇清, 蔡淦. (2005) 中药复方治疗糖尿病肾病的临床研究. 深圳中西医结合杂志 **15**(5): 288–289, 292.
H225	周硕果. (2006) 益气养阴活血法治疗早期糖尿病肾病 40 例临床观察. 中医药临床杂志 **18**(3): 258–259.
H226	朱善勇, 钱才凤. (2013) 蒲参胶囊治疗早期糖尿病肾病的临床疗效观察. 中成药 **35**(4): 681–682.

(*Continued*)

(Continued)

Study Number	References
H227	陈倩倩, 宋宗良. (2013) 益肾活血汤对糖尿病肾病的临床观察. 黑龙江中医药 **5**: 28–29.
H228	董盛, 樊平, 雷根平, 梁瑜, 王婷婷. (2010) 自拟益肾降糖方治疗早期糖尿病肾病临床观察. 中华中医药学刊 **28**(9): 2013–2014.
H229	郭亚平. (2014) 温阳健脾活血中药治疗早期糖尿病肾病脾肾阳虚证临床研究. 中医学报 **29**(7): 965–966.
H230	寇玮蔚, 张明飞. (2014) 清心莲子饮加减治疗早期糖尿病肾病 50 例临床观察. 中国伤残医学 **9**: 167–168.
H231	邝秀英. (2006) 益气养阴活血通腑法联合降糖治疗糖尿病肾病早期的观察. 广东医学 **27**(7): 1096–1098.
H232	林培坚. (2011) 黄芪知母参七颗粒治疗气阴两虚型糖尿病肾病III期临床疗效观察. 福建中医药大学. 学位论文.
H233	牛瑾玉. (2005) 健脾益肾合剂治疗糖尿病肾病 30 例. 陕西中医 **26**(12): 1283–1284.
H234	王姝文. (2008) 参芪降糖颗粒治疗早期糖尿病肾病疗效观察. 辽宁中医杂志 **35**(11): 1710.
H235	代芳. (2014) 调肝补肾活血法合缬沙坦治疗早期糖尿病肾病的临床疗效观察. 山东中医药大学. 学位论文.
H236	郭亚芳, 叶伟成, 曾艺鹏, 唐斌, 王华. (2013) 鹿茸方对早期糖尿病肾病患者 ACR 及转化生长因子-β1 的影响. 新中医 **45**(11): 82–84.
H237	胡连海, 刘文清, 张继东. (2006) 肾康饮治疗早期糖尿病肾病的临床观察及其对患者基质金属蛋白酶-9 水平的影响. 中国中西医结合肾病杂志 **7**(6): 345–346.
H238	秦艳, 庞秀花. (2012) 补肾活血方治疗早期糖尿病肾病 39 例. 中国实验方剂学杂志 **18**(15): 311–313.
H239	武楠, 闫镛, 顾娟娟. (2013) 复方血栓通胶囊联合缬沙坦治疗糖尿病肾病的临床观察. 中国卫生产业: 68, 70.
H240	吴兆芳. (2008) 厄贝沙坦, 金水宝治疗糖尿病肾病临床观察. 实用糖尿病杂志 **4**(6): 18–19.
H241	于海涛, 施海涛, 肖丽丽, 董春玲. (2013) 金水宝联合奥美沙坦酯治疗早期2型糖尿病肾病疗效观察. 当代医学 **19**(23): 64–65.
H242	朱铭卿, 夏佳燕. (2014) 加味当归芍药散联合厄贝沙坦对早期糖尿病肾病患者炎性因子的影响. 中国基层医药 **21**(16): 2546–2547.
H243	曹和欣, 何立群, 黄迪. (2010) 糖肾宁结合西医常规疗法治疗气阴两虚型早期糖尿病肾病 35 例. 上海中医药杂志 **44**(6): 65–67.

(Continued)

(*Continued*)

Study Number	References
H244	邓宝华, 陈忠伟, 王国华, 李雪珍. (2009) 柔肝健脾益肾活血法防治早期糖尿病肾病 34 例临床观察. 山东中医杂志 **28**(3): 156–158.
H245	邓小敏, 唐爱华, 周卫惠. (2006) 培哚普利合用六味地黄丸治疗早期糖尿病肾病的临床疗效观察. 四川中医 **24**(8): 52–53.
H246	邓小敏, 李晶晶, 唐爱华. (2007) 加用参芪地黄汤化裁治疗早期糖尿病肾病临床研究. 广西中医药 **30**(4): 8–10.
H247	窦晨辉, 王松珍. (2014) 黄芪片联合缬沙坦治疗早期糖尿病肾病 24 例. 中医研究 **27**(2): 29–31.
H248	方朝晖, 赵进东. (2012) 苁归益肾胶囊治疗早期糖尿病肾病 60 例临床观察. 中医药临床杂志 **24**(2): 124–125.
H249	冯艳梅. (2011) 益气养阴化瘀通络法治疗 2 型糖尿病肾病III期的临床观察. 黑龙江大学. 学位论文.
H250	洪炜鸿. (2013) 壮肾固精方对糖尿病肾病III期患者尿微量白蛋白的影响. 广州中医药大学. 学位论文.
H251	黄明辉, 甘小斌, 陈建生, 吴端义, 黄舒婕. (2009) "肾康I方"对气阴虚型糖尿病肾病 UMA 的干预作用. 中国中西医结合肾病杂志 **10**(12): 1096.
H252	吉桂萍, 吴景连. (2007) 血脂康胶囊治疗早期糖尿病肾病 32 例. 中国厂矿医学 **20**(3): 226–227.
H253	李荣华. (2014) 益气养阴, 清热解毒, 活血化瘀中药联合洛丁新对早期糖尿病肾病的疗效观察. 山东中医药大学. 学位论文.
H254	廖春才. (2011) 补肾益气法治疗早期糖尿病肾病蛋白尿的临床观察. 北京中医药大学. 学位论文.
H255	林国彬, 叶仁群, 邓淑玲, 曾纪斌, 潘艳, 彭俊杰, 宋群利, 杨丛意. (2011) 补阳还五汤对早期糖尿病肾病患者血清 C-反应蛋白及 PAI-1 的影响. 广州中医药大学学报 **28**(3): 219–221.
H256	刘俊丽. (2014) 降糖平肾方治疗糖尿病肾病（III期）的临床观察. 山东中医药大学. 学位论文.
H257	刘建平, 杨怀书. (2007) 参芪益肾汤治疗早期糖尿病肾病 35 例疗效观察. 中国医药导报 **4**(27): 80–81.
H258	刘立昌, 刘新, 冯敏坚, 张玉婷, 杜雪飞. (2012) 壮肾固精方治疗糖尿病肾病III期的疗效观察. 西部中医药 **25**(4): 11–12.
H259	刘亚丽. (2003) 中西医结合治疗糖尿病早期肾病的临床观察. 山西中医 **19**(5): 29–30.

(*Continued*)

(Continued)

Study Number	References
H260	楼天红, 李晖云, 于磊. (2014) 糖脉康片治疗早期糖尿病肾病的临床疗效及对氧化应激的影响. 新中医 **46**(5): 145–148.
H261	潘桂英, 李登宇, 马莉. (2012) 中西医结合治疗早期糖尿病肾病临床观察. 世界中西医结合杂志 **7**(4): 332–333, 357.
H262	沈蓓莉. (2005) 慢肾宁合剂与洛汀新联合治疗糖尿病肾病微量白蛋白尿的临床观察. 中国中西医结合肾病杂志 **6**(3): 162–163.
H263	沈璐. (2006) 丹芪地黄汤治疗气阴两虚型糖尿病肾病临床研究. 陕西中医药大学. 学位论文.
H264	孙富华, 赵秀娟, 李连英. (2014) 糖肾 I 号治疗糖尿病合并尿蛋白有效性和安全性的临床研究. 辽宁中医杂志 **41**(2): 271–273.
H265	唐咸玉, 朱章志, 陈利平. (2009) 温肾健脾, 祛毒活血法对早期糖尿病肾病及 IL-6, TNF-α 的影响. 中药新药与临床药理 **20**(2): 175–177.
H266	王国庆, 安金龙, 俞仲贤, 张雪峰, 张文军, 金仲达. (2014) 加减滋膵饮联合厄贝沙坦治疗III期糖尿病肾病的临床观察. 内蒙古中医药 **33**(9): 25–26
H267	王化鹏. (2007) 福辛普利联用金水宝治疗早期 2 型糖尿病肾病临床观察. 天津药学 **19**(3): 27–28.
H268	王萍. (2010) 脑心通联合缬沙坦治疗高血压并发糖尿病早期肾损害疗效观察. 中医临床研究 **2**(21): 40–41.
H269	王兴民, 季海峰, 叶方益. (2009) 中药辅助治疗 2 型糖尿病早期肾病 24 例. 浙江中西医结合杂志 **19**(3): 161–162.
H270	吴刚花, 张小平. (2005) 中西医结合治疗早期糖尿病肾病 30 例临床观察. 中医药导报 **11**(5): 23–24.
H271	徐芝秀. (2013) 益气养阴中药治疗糖尿肾病临床 60 例疗效观察·海峡药学 **25**(4): 159–160.
H272	闫香梅. (2011) 中药治疗糖尿病肾病 58 例临床分析. 中国社区医师·医学专业 **13**(21): 189.
H273	叶彬华, 钟索娅, 张政, 阮诗玮. (2014) 益肾降糖饮治疗糖尿病肾病III期气阴两虚夹瘀疗效及舌象观察 30 例. 中国中医药现代远程教育 **12**(5): 45–47.
H274	余晓琳, 陈军平, 林晨, 陈敏, 周强, 邱东峰, 黄琛, 黄胜. (2012) 益气活血汤对早期糖尿病肾病患者微量白蛋白尿, 超敏 C 反应蛋白的影响. 光明中医 **27**(9): 1800–1802.
H275	云鹏, 龚婷, 马玲, 肖虎. (2013) 氯沙坦联合复方血栓通胶囊治疗早期糖尿病肾病的临床研究. 中国现代医学杂志 **23**(4): 67–70.

(Continued)

(Continued)

Study Number	References
H276	曾纪斌, 杨越, 甘斌, 宋晓容, 于月明, 辛俊平, 傅诗书. (2008) 鹿茸丸治疗早期糖尿病肾病 60 例的临床观察. 世界中医药 **3**(1): 15–17.
H277	张彩萍, 刘金耀. (2011) 中西医结合治疗早期糖尿病肾病 40 例临床观察. 浙江中医杂志 **46**(4): 277–278.
H278	张丹芳, 程时杰. (2009) 自拟固肾健脾方治疗糖尿病III期肾病 28 例. 江西中医药 **40**(6): 28–29.
H279	张海生, 薛京花. (2010) 糖肾方治疗早期糖尿病肾病 36 例. 中国民间疗法 **18**(4): 32–33.
H280	章九红, 李文泉, 耿建国, 杜宇琼, 苗力, 邢兆宏, 张铖. (2015) 加味消渴康治疗糖尿病肾病临床疗效观察. 北京中医药 **34**(1): 42895.
H281	赵海彬, 梁晴, 徐鹏飞. (2008) 疏糖益肾丸治疗糖尿病肾病临床观察. 现代中西医结合杂志 **17**(23): 3600–3601.
H282	赵明刚, 马茂芝. (2014) 益气温阳化瘀法治疗早期糖尿病肾病临床研究. 山东中医杂志 **33**(2): 99–100.
H283	钟宏琳. (2004) 依那普利与通塞脉联合治疗糖尿病肾病疗效观察. 医学文选 **23**(5): 602.
H284	鲍普强. (2014) 葛芪降糖颗粒治疗早期糖尿病肾病的临床研究. 北京中医药大学. 学位论文.
H285	蔡庆春, 李小冰, 樊学忠, 闫利利. (2006) 水蛭通胶囊对早期糖尿病肾病患者血脂血流变的影响. 中国中医药信息杂志 **13**(7): 67–68.
H286	曹雪霞, 张鹏睿, 杨金奎. (2007) 金水宝联合缬沙坦治疗2型糖尿病肾病的早期疗效. 中国新药杂志 **16**(16): 1303–1306.
H287	陈翠兰, 张兴坤, 车树强. (2014) 糖肾康胶囊对糖尿病肾病III期尿微量白蛋白的影响. 天津中医药 **31**(10): 596–598.
H288	陈永斌, 万永富. (2011) 芪参益气滴丸治疗 2 型糖尿病早期肾病的疗效研究. 中国全科医学 **14**(2B): 520–522.
H289	范一超, 祝全. (2009) 中西医结合治疗早期糖尿病肾病 28 例临床观察. 江苏中医药 **41**(7): 41–42.
H290	范一超, 陆新, 施爱华. (2014) 中西医结合治疗早期糖尿病肾病 60 例临床观察. 江苏中医药 **46**(7): 38–39.
H291	方朝晖, 程森华, 吴倩. (2013) 丹蛭降糖胶囊对早期糖尿病肾病患者血 NF-κB 和尿白蛋白排泄率的影响. 世界科学技术·中医药现代化 **15**(5): 891–895.

(Continued)

(Continued)

Study Number	References
H292	冯天保, 陈刚毅, 谢桂权. (2005) 康肾汤治疗早期糖尿病肾病的临床观察. 湖北中医杂志 **27**(9): 17–19.
H293	高祥. (2011) 血塞通软胶囊联合替米沙坦治疗早期糖尿病肾病临床观察. 医学信息: 中旬刊 (5): 2065–2066.
H294	葛其容. (2011) 盐酸贝那普利联合金水宝胶囊治疗糖尿病肾病的疗效观察. 中国卫生产业 **8**(7): 59.
H295	宫晶书, 王和天. (2004) 养阴益气合剂治疗早期糖尿病肾病临床观察. 中药研究与信息 **6**(8): 18–19.
H296	古青. (2008) 通心络胶囊联合开博通对早期糖尿病肾病尿微量白蛋白的影响. 疑难病杂志 **7**(10): 606–607.
H297	郭成坤, 张琴. (2012) 葫芦巴联合缬沙坦治疗糖尿病肾病的疗效观察. 疑难病杂志 **11**(3): 191–193.
H298	季兵, 关健华, 陈先明, 谢政权, 林靖, 高飞. (2012) 自拟补肾活血方治疗早期糖尿病肾病40例临床观察. 当代医学 **18**(10): 1–2.
H299	金晟. (2014) 滋阴活血法联合缬沙坦治疗早期糖尿病肾病的临床观察. 湖北中医药大学学报 **16**(5): 61–63.
H300	康善平, 彭绍杰. (2008) 益气活血法治疗老年早期糖尿病肾病的疗效观察. 辽宁中医药大学学报 **10**(7): 3–4.
H301	李宝纯, 刘树文, 李青. (2009) 补阳还五汤治疗III期糖尿病肾病 102 例临床观察. 中国中医药科技 **16**(2): 142–143.
H302	李劲松. (2009) 益气健脾补肾活血法治疗早期糖尿病肾病 33 例. 福建中医药 **40**(5): 35–36.
H303	李性周. (2005) 红参虫草胶囊对早期糖尿病肾病的临床治疗作用. 延边大学. 学位论文.
H304	李志强, 常红娟, 孙仕润. (2013) 自拟益气活血方治疗糖尿病肾病疗效以及对血液流变学和相关生化指标的影响. 中国中医基础医学杂志 **19**(6): 657–659.
H305	廖欣, 王海燕, 王祚邦, 辛俊平, 宋晓容, 叶仁群, 刘成彬. (2011) 六味地黄加味方治疗早期糖尿病肾病临床研究. 中国中医药信息杂志 **18**(9): 13–15.
H306	林跃辉, 嵇美霞, 胡岗, 黄培荣. (2010) 加味参芪地黄汤辅助治疗糖尿病肾病临床观察. 浙江中西医结合杂志 **20**(11): 679–680.
H307	刘凤环, 蔡厚田, 王秀玲. (2005) 糖肾康胶囊治疗早期糖尿病肾病临床观察. 河南中医 **25**(2): 45–46.

(Continued)

(Continued)

Study Number	References
H308	罗红艳. (2008) 补肾活血方治疗早期糖尿病肾病的临床研究. 科学技术与工程 **8**(8): 2176–2179.
H309	吕洪, 刘静芹, 贾振祥, 何红梅. (2006) 金水宝与缬沙坦联合治疗早期糖尿病肾病的疗效观察. 中国医师杂志: 291–292.
H310	牛云飞, 方朝晖, 刘剑, 石国斌. (2008) 丹蛭降糖胶囊治疗老年糖尿病早期肾病的临床研究. 中国现代中药 **10**(5): 36–38.
H311	潘艳伶, 凌湘力. (2015) 糖通饮对早期糖尿病肾病患者尿微量白蛋白排泄率, 糖脂代谢的影响. 北方药学 **12**(2): 112–113.
H312	庞韬, 李新华. (2014) 通络固肾丸治疗 2 型糖尿病肾病III期的临床疗效观察. 第十五次全国中医糖尿病大会: 334–339.
H313	乔爱民. (2013) 替米沙坦联合百令胶囊治疗早期糖尿病肾病 62 例疗效观察. 中国实用医药 **8**(28): 177–178.
H314	邱晓堂, 张永杰, 吴中虎, 霍娟勇, 高伟铿, 王巧凡. (2007) 滋脾通络汤治疗糖尿病早期肾病临床观察. 中华中医药学刊 **25**(6): 1169–1171.
H315	屈岭, 王祥生, 曹爱国. (2011) 灵芝健肾胶囊对糖尿病肾病血脂和血流动力学的影响. 甘肃中医 **24**(1): 28–30.
H316	沈生妹. (2012) 缬沙坦联合百令胶囊治疗早期糖尿病肾病 86 例疗效观察. 中国基层医药 **19**(1): 127–128.
H317	施维敏. (2012) 糖肾康饮治疗早期 2 型糖尿病肾病气阴两虚夹瘀型的临床研究. 黑龙江中医药大学. 学位论文.
H318	唐通, 王聪. (2006) 活血祛湿法治疗早期糖尿病肾病的疗效观察. 中华实用中西医杂志 **19**(24): 2911–2912.
H319	王培红, 陈晓丽. (2005) 自拟糖肾康汤治疗早期糖尿病肾病的临床观察. 山西医药杂志 **34**(10): 873–874.
H320	王文凤, 黄庆仪, 赖小菊. (2008) 中西医结合治疗早期糖尿病肾病临床研究. 河南中医学院学报 **23**(6): 44–45.
H321	王欣, 田伟伟, 安丽萍. (2013) 自拟黄蛭方治疗早期糖尿病肾病临床研究. 四川中医 **31**(2): 70–72.
H322	王学玲, 张平. (2012) 灯盏生脉胶囊联合依那普利治疗 2 型糖尿病早期肾病的临床研究. 中国实用医药 **7**(27): 8–10.
H323	王运红, 袁桂芬. (2008) 百令胶囊联合替米沙坦治疗早期糖尿病肾病的临床观察. 医学临床研究 **25**(5): 927–928.
H324	魏罡杰. (2010) 糖脂平治疗糖尿病微血管并发症早期糖尿病肾病的临床研究. 黑龙江中医药大学. 学位论文.

(Continued)

(Continued)

Study Number	References
H325	吴文霞. (2010) 健脾补肾化瘀通络方联合西药治疗早期糖尿病肾病 30 例. 中医药临床杂志 (6): 476–477.
H326	徐婷芳. (2014) 五子衍宗丸加味方治疗脾肾亏虚兼瘀证 3 期糖尿病肾病的疗效研究. 福建中医药大学. 学位论文.
H327	杨娜, 张德宪. (2011) 金匮肾气丸结合洛丁新治疗阴阳两虚型糖尿病肾病临床观察. 山东中医药大学学报 **35**(3): 232–234.
H328	杨朔. (2007) 糖肾平方配合苯那普利治疗气阴两虚夹瘀型早期 2 型糖尿病肾病的临床研究. 福建中医学院. 学位论文.
H329	岳超, 曹龙宇, 赵丹阳. (2007) 中西医结合治疗早期糖尿病肾病的临床研究. 中医药学报 **35**(1): 60–62.
H330	张庚良. (2012) 益气养阴活血方治疗早期糖尿病肾病 40 例临床观察. 河北中医 **34**(6): 829–830.
H331	张海男, 胡随瑜, 李云辉. (2005) 中西医结合治疗早期 2 型糖尿病肾病的临床观察. 湖南中医学院学报 **25**(6): 45–47.
H332	张惠珍, 张慎友, 董林. (1999) 糖肾胶囊治疗早期糖尿病肾病临床研究. 北京中医 (6): 17–18.
H333	张丽丽. (2008) 糖肾康饮治疗气阴两虚夹瘀型 2 型糖尿病早期肾病的临床研究. 黑龙江中医药大学. 学位论文.
H334	张硕. (2010) 益肾化浊汤治疗（肾阴亏虚, 瘀浊互结证）早期糖尿病肾病（III期）的临床观察. 长春中医药大学. 学位论文.
H335	张众. (2004) 糖肾康治疗早期糖尿病肾病疗效观察. 四川中医 (5): 42–43.
H336	郑作孜. (2005) 六味地黄汤加减治疗早期糖尿病肾病微量白蛋白尿之临床观察. 湖北中医学院. 学位论文.
H337	周玉莲. (2014) 运用施今墨药对治疗早期糖尿病肾病的疗效观察. 世界中医药 **9**(5): 574–576.
H338	朱善勇. (2010) 健脾益肾清利通络法治疗早期糖尿病肾病的临床研究. 南京中医药大学. 学位论文.
H339	杜珍芳, 强胜, 黄敏, 翟惟凯. (2013) 益气养阴通络法治疗 3 期糖尿病肾病 30 例. 河南中医 **33**(12): 2123–2124.
H340	李萍, 韩阳. (2013) 自拟运脾益肾活络汤治疗糖尿病肾病疗效评价. 中国中西医结合急救杂志 **20**(1): 39–41.
H341	李雪珍. (2010) 活血化瘀法治疗糖尿病肾病临床观察. 中医临床研究 **2**(22): 40.

(Continued)

(**Continued**)

Study Number	References
H342	刘克冕, 王小超, 狄红杰, 谢绍峰. (2009) 消渴肾康汤联合贝那普利治疗早期糖尿病肾病临床研究. 实用中医药杂志 **25**(1): 26–27.
H343	肖荣. (2014) 益气养血, 通络消积法治疗糖尿病肾病III期的临床研究. 山东中医药大学. 学位论文.
H344	于晓瑜, 蒙向欣, 赵威. (2014) 加味芪黄饮治疗早期糖尿病肾病临床研究. 黑龙江中医药 (2): 30–31.
H345	赵文霞, 刘学芬. (2011) 益肾灵汤剂降低早期糖尿病肾病患者尿微量白蛋白的临床观察. 现代中西医结合杂志 **20**(8): 972–973.
H346	蔡然. (2014) 中西医结合治疗早期糖尿病肾病 30 例临床观察. 中医药导报 **20**(16): 66–68.
H347	陈辉, 汤水福, 赵萍. (2005) 活血化瘀法治疗早期糖尿病肾病及其对肾血流参数的影响. 中国中西医结合肾病杂志 **6**(1): 31–32.
H348	李先行, 刘爱华. (2012) 升清降浊方治疗糖尿病肾病III期蛋白尿 30 例. 中国中医药现代远程教育 **10**(17): 16–17.
H349	刘成彬. (2011) 益气养阴祛湿通络法对早期糖尿病肾病的疗效观察. 广州中医药大学. 学位论文.
H350	宋宗良, 张璇. (2009) 益肾活血方治疗早期糖尿病肾病 46 例临床观察. 辽宁中医杂志 **36**(8): 1337–1338.
H351	孙新宇, 武西芳, 高大红. (2012) 解毒通络法对早期糖尿病肾病炎症发病机制的干预研究. 中国中医基础医学杂志 **18**(5): 527–528.
H352	王天平. (2014) 金水宝联合依那普利治疗糖尿病肾病随机平行对照研究. 实用中医内科杂志 **28**(11): 77–79.
H353	吴丽娜. (2010) 中西医结合治疗早期糖尿病肾病临床观察. 辽宁医学院学报 **31**(1): 59–60.
H354	叶仁群, 林国彬, 邓淑玲, 增纪斌, 潘艳, 彭俊杰, 宋群利, 杨丛意. (2011) 补阳还五汤对早期糖尿病肾病患者血清白细胞介素-6 及肿瘤坏死因子-α 的影响. 河北中医 **33**(3): 383–385.
H355	原守平. (2015) 缬沙坦联合复方地龙胶囊治疗对早期糖尿病肾病患者尿蛋白总量的影响. 福建医药杂志 **37**(1): 90–92.
H356	陈志强, 郭登洲, 孙玉凤, 檀金川, 王月华. (2008) 益气养阴消癥通络中药治疗糖尿病肾病临床观察. 中医药学会肾病分会学术会议论文: 165–167.
H357	丁艳, 李性周, 崔海月, 赵贤俊. (2004) 解毒保肾汤治疗早期糖尿病性肾病. 延边大学医学学报 **27**(1): 45–48.

(*Continued*)

(Continued)

Study Number	References
H358	范冠杰, 黎永富, 唐爱华, 李双蕾, 李晶晶, 罗广波, 周卫惠. (2007) 止消保肾汤对早期糖尿病肾病 NO 及 SOD 的影响. 北京中医药大学学报 **30**(3): 210–212.
H359	冯志海. (2002) 玉液汤加减治疗早期糖尿病肾病 36 例临床观察. 中国医药学报 **17**(9): 539–540.
H360	郭登洲, 王月华, 张芬芳, 王彦凯, 陈志强. (2007) 活血化淤消瘀通络中药治疗糖尿病肾病 76 例临床研究. 中国全科医学 **10**(20): 1692–1693.
H361	李红专. (2006) 糖肾宁对早期糖尿病肾病患者肾功能保护作用的临床研究. 山东大学. 学位论文.
H362	李淑彦, 宋维明, 杨露梅, 李青, 朱钰宝. (2010) 滋肾固精凉血法对早期糖尿病肾病尿微量白蛋白的影响. 国际中医中药杂志 **32**(2): 115–116.
H363	李彦芬, 周新灵, 陈伟. (2013) 益气通络保肾汤对糖尿病肾病疗效的观察. 河北中医 **35**(12): 1798–1799.
H364	李玉忠, 孔祥英, 卢笑辉. (2005) 补肾固精法治疗早期糖尿病肾病 60 例. 山东中医药大学学报 **29**(4): 289–290.
H365	刘可. (2003) 盘消 4 号片治疗早期糖尿病肾病的临床研究. 中国中医药科技 **10**(3): 134–135.
H366	任国英. (2008) 自拟糖肾安汤治疗早期糖尿病肾病 35 例临床观察. 实用中医内科杂志 (5): 44–45.
H367	唐晨光, 莫新民. (2009) 消渴漏微煎治疗早期糖尿病肾病的临床观察. 深圳中西医结合杂志 **19**(2): 112–114.
H368	佟杰, 杨荣阁. (2011) 益气活血渗湿泄浊法治疗早期糖尿病肾病临床观察. 河北中医 **33**(1): 53–54.
H369	王志萍, 刘利平, 王彦丽, 马毓. (2008) 糖肾消饮治疗早期糖尿病肾病疗效观察. 中国中医急症 **17**(4): 466–467.
H370	吴瑞, 崔文旺. (2013) 益气养阴活血方治疗早期糖尿病肾病 30 例. 河南中医 **33**(11): 1923–1924.
H371	许粤. (2004) 以往一般用补液, 参芪活血汤治疗早期糖尿病肾病变. 中华实用中西医杂志 **4**(17): 2617–2618.
H372	张波, 秦佰焰. (2012) 济生肾气丸联合复方血栓通胶囊治疗早期糖尿病肾病. 中国实验方剂学杂志 **18**(15): 316–317.
H373	张丽萍. (2012) 益气养阴, 解毒活血法对早期糖尿病肾病 D-二聚体, CRP 影响的研究. 北京中医药大学. 学位论文.

(Continued)

(*Continued*)

Study Number	References
H374	张昱, 李琦, 娄锡恩. (2008) 护肾愈消汤治疗早期糖尿病肾病 38 例的临床观察. 世界中医药 **3**(1): 21–22.
H375	安向平, 檀金川, 戴剑华. (2008) 莪黄糖肾合剂对早期糖尿病肾病血脂, 尿白蛋白排泄率及血液流变学的影响. 河北中医 **30**(8): 792–794.
H376	陈景亮, 凌方明. (2004) 六味地黄丸对早期糖尿病肾病尿微量白蛋白的影响. 新中医 **36**(12): 26–27.
H377	董彦敏, 李慧林, 倪青. (2007) 益气活血法治疗糖尿病早期肾病 34 例临床观察. 新中医 **39**(6): 76–78.
H378	冯乐燕. (2005) 固本化瘀消浊法治疗早期糖尿病肾病的临床研究. 山东中医药大学. 学位论文.
H379	何泽, 朴春丽, 黄净, 米佳, 包扬, 李金博. (2015) 消渴肾安胶囊干预早期糖尿病肾病尿微量白蛋白及氧化应激 40 例. 中国中医药现代远程教育 **13**(4): 4–6.
H380	黄延芹, 徐云生. (2008) 补肾活血通络法治疗早期糖尿病肾病 38 例临床观察. 中医杂志 **49**(5): 421–423.
H381	李留霞. (2013) 健脾补肾通络方治疗糖尿病肾病III期 36 例疗效观察. 世界中西医结合杂志 **8**(9): 921–923.
H382	林兰, 倪青, 高齐健, 张润云, 胡东鹏, 刘喜明, 苏诚炼, 陈思兰, 魏军平, 李鸣镝. (2000) 糖微康胶囊治疗糖尿病肾病的临床观察. 中国中西医结合杂志 **20**(11): 811–814.
H383	唐爱华, 周卫惠, 钟金清, 王少柯. (2010) 化浊益肾方对早期糖尿病肾病患者 VEGF 的影响. 辽宁中医药杂志 **38**(1): 107–108. [王少柯. (2010) 化浊益肾方治疗早期糖尿病肾病疗效观察及对患者血清 VEGF 的影响. 广西中医药大学. 学位论文.]
H384	唐晨光, 潘勤, 陈腾云, 黄蕾, 孙海膺, 李雪梅, 梁池莲. (2010) 消渴漏微方治疗早期糖尿病肾病的临床研究. 新中医 **42**(2): 41–43.
H385	唐红, 李红, 徐蓉娟, 葛芳芳, 胡健炜, 杨华. (2001) 益气活血补肾法对早期糖尿病肾病血管活性物质的影响. 上海中医杂志 (12): 19–20.
H386	王刚, 郭晓玲, 魏晓娜, 陈志强, 檀金川. (2006) 糖肾合剂对早期糖尿病肾病患者尿微量白蛋白排泄率及内皮素-1和一氧化氮的影响. 河北中医 **28**(9): 651–653.
H387	王会芳, 张爱旗, 宗克亮. (2011) 益气助肾口服液治疗早期糖尿病肾病 42 例临床观察. 河北中医 **33**(12): 1788–1790.
H388	王文红. (2012) 益气补肾活血汤治疗糖尿病肾病III期35例疗效观察. 光明中医 **27**(12): 2441–2442.

(*Continued*)

(Continued)

Study Number	References
H389	薛婧, 白君伟, 梁苹茂. (2008) 六味地黄汤治疗早期糖尿病肾病 36 例临床观察. 实用中医内科杂志 (2): 31.
H390	薛晓彤, 程益春, 陈建衡. (2007) 糖肾灵治疗早期糖尿病肾病临床研究. 中国中医药信息杂志 **14**(1): 20–22.
H391	姚秀明. (2014) 祛胰抵方治疗早期 2 型糖尿病肾病的临床观察及对尿 CTGF 的影响. 黑龙江中医药大学. 学位论文.
H392	于梅, 迟继铭, 张岩岩, 姜国华. (2012) 肾炎消白颗粒对早期糖尿病肾病患者尿白蛋白及血清 TGF-β1 的影响. 中医药信息 **29**(1): 43–44.
H393	张秋梅. (2015) 中西医结合治疗早期糖尿病肾病 50 例观察. 实用中医药杂志 **31**(3): 211–212.
H394	赵学兰, 邱召运, 王金玲, 王燕, 史红霞. (2007) 苯那普利与黄芪当归合剂治疗糖尿病肾病临床观察. 临床荟萃 (2): 131–132.
H395	祁燕, 孙晓红. (2013) 复方固肾冲剂和蒙诺片治疗老年糖尿病肾病肾虚血瘀型蛋白尿临床对比分析. 大家健康(学术版) **7**(8): 58.
H396	徐英. (2005) 保肾汤治疗早期糖尿病肾病 32 例. 辽宁中医杂志 **32**(3): 213.
H397	曹松华. (2010) 中西医结合治疗早期糖尿病肾病 32 例疗效观察. 国医论坛 **25**(6): 35–36.
H398	陈彤君, 徐晖. (2013) 健脾通络方对早期糖尿病肾病微量白蛋白尿排泄率的影响. 四川中医 **31**(4): 69–70.
H399	郭玉洁. (2007) 复方丹参滴丸治疗早期糖尿病肾病的临床观察. 中国民康医学 **19**(2): 117–118.
H400	安玲, 董军梅, 牛振霞. (2009) 糖肾康胶囊治疗早期糖尿病肾病 35 例. 世界中医药 **4**(5): 261–262.
H401	陈汉礼, 周茹, 陆标明. (2010) 金水宝胶囊合山楂消脂胶囊对早期糖尿病肾病血浆内皮素Ⅰ及 C 反应蛋白的影响. 湖南中医药大学学报 **30**(6): 35–37.
H402	陈际连, 陈晓雯, 扬升杰, 钱力维, 刘怀珍, 张进军, 李居一. (2013) 复方健胰胶囊治疗早期糖尿病肾病气阴两虚夹痰瘀型疗效观察. 河北中医 **35**(9): 294–296.
H403	翟熙君. (2014) 活血益肾方治疗早期糖尿病肾病临床研究. 中医学报 **29**(8): 1119–1121.
H404	黄静, 姜莉莉, 吴军. (2006) 降糖益肾胶囊治疗早期糖尿病肾病的临床研究. 中国民间疗法 **14**(6): 3–4.

(Continued)

(*Continued*)

Study Number	References
H405	黄静, 邹彦, 薛玲玲. (2007) 降糖活血饮改善早期糖尿病肾病临床观察. 中医药临床杂志 **19**(5): 437–439.
H406	刘香红, 杨晨. (2014) 补肾活血方治疗早期糖尿病肾病蛋白尿 56 例临床观察. 中国中医基础医学杂志 **20**(7): 998–999.
H407	刘渊. (2014) 益气养阴补肾活血方剂治疗早期糖尿病肾病的临床观察. 光明中医 **29**(7): 1392–1394.
H408	陆继敏. (2015) 健脾凉血化瘀汤治疗糖尿病肾病 45 例临床观察. 河北中医 **37**(3): 372–374.
H409	罗崇谦, 潘素滢, 胡桂兴. (2008) 滋肾汤治疗早期糖尿病肾病临床疗效观察. 甘肃中医学院学报 **25**(3): 27–29.
H410	潘满立, 王静飞, 庞秀花. (2014) 益气养阴活血祛湿法治疗早期糖尿病肾病的临床研究. 北京中医药 **33**(2): 134–137.
H411	王宪波, 桑雁, 孔祥梅, 乔立新, 单春光, 韩清. (2007) 糖肾 II 号胶囊合并西药治疗非胰岛素依赖型糖尿病伴微白蛋白尿的临床观察. 中国中西医结合杂志 **17**(10): 622–623.
H412	王艳丽, 宋萌涵, 刁建华. (2013) 芪药消渴胶囊治疗早期糖尿病肾病 41例. 现代中医药 **33**(4): 32–34.
H413	吴松林. (2003) 糖适平片联合丹蒌合剂治疗糖尿病肾病 30 例. 现代中西医结合杂志 **12**(10): 1030–1031.
H414	杨梅, 魏于虹, 徐丽. (2009) 六黄益津丸对糖尿病肾病及代谢多因素干预的临床研究. 医学研究与教育 **26**(3): 72–73.
H415	张晶晶. (2011) 糖脉康颗粒治疗早期糖尿病肾病蛋白尿的临床观察. 广州中医药大学. 学位论文.
H416	张文学. (2010) 益肾合剂治疗糖尿病早期肾病 30 例临床观察. 中国社区医师·医学专业 **12**(18): 136–137.
H417	赵郴, 马中建, 陈玉林, 罗学林. (2008) 尿毒清颗粒对早期糖尿病肾病 68例疗效观察. 中国医学创新 **5**(36): 145–147.
H418	郑鹏哲, 陈琪. (2014) 健脾温肾汤治疗糖尿病肾病 40 例临床观察. 浙江中医杂志 **49**(3): 185.
H419	朱银花, 魏棠, 刘晋熹. (2006) 益气活血保肾解毒法治疗早期糖尿病肾病 30 例. 中国民间疗法 **14**(6): 6–7.
H420	李军. (2007) 中西医结合治疗对早期糖尿病肾病尿微量白蛋白影响的临床观察. 中华中医药学刊 **25**(6): 1302–1304.

(*Continued*)

(*Continued*)

Study Number	References
H421	唐红, 李红, 徐蓉娟, 杨华, 葛芳芳, 宋怡萍. (2005) 治糖保肾冲剂调控血小板衍化生长因子-β 逆转早期糖尿病肾病机制的临床研究. 上海中医药杂志 **39**(11): 29–30.
H422	徐坤英. (2006) 自拟芪贞六味益肾饮治疗早期糖尿病肾病的临床观察. 北京中医 **25**(8): 480–481.
H423	钟成福, 刘旭阳, 周雪, 张志华, 刘佳. (2010) 小剂量螺内酯联合复方丹参滴丸治疗早期糖尿病肾病尿白蛋白的疗效观察. 临床荟萃 **25**(10): 898–900.
H424	栗瑶. (2012) 百令胶囊治疗早期糖尿病肾病的临床观察. 中国社区医师·医学专业 **14**(5): 185.
H425	李斌. (2004) 中西医结合治疗早期糖尿病肾病 20 例小结. 湖南中医药导报 **10**(7): 16–17.
H426	高彦彬, 吕仁和, 王秀琴, 庚及第, 任可, 王越, 赵进喜, 于秀辰, 陈丁生. (1997) 糖肾宁治疗糖尿病肾病的临床研究. 中医杂志 **38**(2): 96–99.
H427	陈化龙, 沙一岭, 李福东. (2008) 活血化瘀法治疗糖尿病肾病 36 例临床观察. 中国煤炭工业医学杂志 **11**(5): 752.
H428	陈逢春, 张效科. (2014) 消渴方加减联合马来酸依那普利治疗早期DN的疗效观察. 健康导报: 医学版 **12**(19): 119.
H429	彭卫华, 曲强, 陈建. (2000) 血脂康对合并高脂血症的 2 型糖尿病患者微量蛋白尿的影响. 福州总医院学报 **7**(4): 17–19.
H430	张阳, 邓志斌, 李萍. (2004) 血脂康对合并高脂血症的 2 型糖尿病患者微量白蛋白尿的影响. 中国医学研究与临床 **2**(1): 29–30.
H431	赵章华. (2009) 益气养阴化瘀汤对早期糖尿病肾病患者超敏 C 反应蛋白, 内皮素-1 和尿微量蛋白排泄率的影响. 中医研究 (10): 37–39.
H432	Ma J, Xu L, Dong J, Wei H, Zhi Y, Ma X, Zhang X. (2013) Effects of Zishentongluo in Patients. *Am J Chin Med* **41**(2): 333–340.
H433	黄柳莺, 张娟娟. (2011) 中药肾区离子导入治疗糖尿病肾病的临床观察. 中国现代药物应用 **5**(20): 52–53.
H434	戴舜珍, 苏小惠. (2005) 中西医结合治疗早期糖尿病肾病临床观察. 辽宁中医杂志 **32**(12): 1289–1290.
H435	周兰, 姚诗清, 柳雯, 孙涛, 汪超, 陈莉. (2015) 芪藿复方合剂联合西药治疗糖尿病肾病III期临床研究. 安徽中医药大学学报 **34**(22): 33–36.

(*Continued*)

(*Continued*)

Study Number	References
H436	杨福新, 苏秀海, 李烨. (2000) 糖肾宁治疗早期糖尿病肾病临床观察. 全国第六次中医糖尿病学术会议: 294–296.
H437	谢甦, 凌湘力. (2011) 糖通饮对早期糖尿病肾病尿白蛋白肌酐比值血液流变学的影响. 福建中医药大学学报 **21**(2): 8–10.
H438	毛春谱, 李小毅, 李伟. (2010) 参芪降糖颗粒对早期糖尿病肾病患者血清 TGF-β1, VEGF 的影响. 第三军医大学学报 **32**(13): 1475–1476.
H439	沈晓明, 江艳, 徐雪根. (2010) 银杏叶片辅助治疗早期糖尿病肾病疗效观察. 中国医师杂志 **12**(5): 696–697.
H440	黄菊, 陈风和. (2013) 中药足浴辅助治疗糖尿病肾病的疗效观察. 中南医学科学杂志 **41**(6): 647–649.
H441	田佳星, 赵林华, 周强, 仝小林. (2012) 抵当汤加减治疗糖尿病肾病微量蛋白尿的回顾性分析. 北京中医药大学学报·中医临床版 **19**(6): 7–10.
H442	冯兴中, 姜敏, 卢苇, 周铭. (2011) 固肾解毒法治疗糖尿病肾病早期的临床观察. 北京中医药大学学报 **34**(4): 286–288.
H443	冯彬, 唐培荣, 王如. (2007) 黄连素治疗早期糖尿病肾病临床疗效观察. 中国当代医学 **6**(9): 72.
H444	文平凡, 黄桂琼. (2011) 黄连四物汤治疗早期糖尿病肾病的临床疗效观察及对血清 ages 水平的影响. 中华中医药学刊 **29**(4): 921–923.
H445	曹永芬. (2007) 中药健脾保肾方治疗老年人早期糖尿病肾病的临床观察. 辽宁中医杂志 (9): 1267.
H446	白英秀. (2007) 糖肾安治疗早期糖尿病肾病 60 例临床观察. 光明中医 **22**(10): 79–80.
H447	马彩云, 孙西霞, 翟哲. (2010) 通心络胶囊联合缬沙坦胶囊治疗 2 型糖尿病肾病 125 例. 现代中西医结合杂志 **19**(22): 2789–2790.
H448	马彩云, 孙西霞, 翟哲. (2009) 缬沙坦联合通心络治疗糖尿病肾病的临床观察. 中国医学创新 **6**(22): 83–84.
H449	曹和欣, 何立群, 侯卫国, 邹世林. (2006) 糖肾宁对早中期糖尿病肾病患者蛋白尿的作用及机理研究. 中华中医药学会第十九次全国中医肾病学术交流会: 89–93.
H450	张丽萍, 娄锡恩, 高晶. (2012) 娄锡恩教授治疗早期糖尿病肾病的临床经验. 四川中医 **30**(5): 3–5.
H451	詹锐文, 邹宁. (2004) 早肾方联合卡托普利治疗早期糖尿病肾病的临床研究. 河北中医 (11): 811–812.

(*Continued*)

(Continued)

Study Number	References
H452	张惠. (2010) 益气活血补肾法治疗糖尿病早期肾病 35 例. 实用中医内科杂志 **24**(4): 58.
H453	孔凡俊. (2011) 中西医结合治疗早期糖尿病肾病 50 例临床观察. 实用中西医结合临床 **11**(2): 26–27.
H454	阳晓, 阳旭. (2004) 中西医结合治疗早期糖尿病肾病的疗效观察. 中国实用乡村医生杂志 **11**(11): 28–29.
H455	罗苏生, 泮如琴, 郑翠瑛, 汪隽芳, 叶美颜. (1993) 补肾活血法治疗糖尿病早期肾病. 浙江中医学院学报 **17**(6): 12.
H456	谢晓月. (2011) 王镁教授补脾法治疗糖尿病肾病经验总结. 辽宁中医药大学. 学位论文.
H457	宋雪娟. (2012) 黄葵胶囊治疗早期糖尿病肾病的疗效观察. 吉林医学 **33**(29): 6333–6334.
H458	姜玉环, 李明霞. (2008) 卡托普利和血塞通胶囊治疗早期糖尿病肾病临床观察. 医学创新研究 **5**(17): 150–151.
H459	许珍, 王淑玲. (2004) 疏肝补肾益气中药对早期糖尿病肾病患者 ei-1 及 cgrp 的影响. 中国中西医结合肾病杂志 **5**(10): 609–610.
H460	朱丽光. (2008) 糖尿病肾病验案三则. 天津中医药 **25**(3): 253.
H461	高思博. (2014) 消渴肾病方治疗糖尿病肾病 3 期气阴两虚,痰瘀互结型的临床观察. 黑龙江中医药大学. 学位论文.
H462	徐蓉娟, 唐红, 胡健炜, 钟家宝. (1995) 益肾宝治疗肾阴亏虚型早期糖尿病肾病 34 例临床观察. 上海中医药大学学报 **9**(2): 31–33.
H463	常淑玲. (2002) 自拟益肾汤治疗早期糖尿病肾病 40 例临床观察. 北京中医 **21**(4): 225–226.
H464	吕蕾. (1999) 中西医结合治疗 II 型糖尿病早期肾病 30 例临床疗效观察. 中医药研究 **15**(3): 32–33.

6

Pharmacological Actions of Frequently Used Herbs and Formulas

OVERVIEW

Chinese herbal medicines and their constituent compounds may improve diabetic kidney disease (DKD) by reducing free radical damage, inflammation and mesangial matrix expansion of the kidney. To explain the possible biological activity of the frequently used Chinese herbs, this chapter reviews the experimental evidence and provides a summary of their mechanisms of action relevant to the pathophysiological processes of DKD.

Introduction

Chinese herbal formulae and herbs exert their actions through active constituent compounds. Experimental evidence, including *in vitro* and *in vivo* studies, helps to explain the possible mechanisms of action of the herbs and how they may improve the signs and symptoms of diabetic kidney disease (DKD). This chapter presents a general overview of the experimental evidence from cell lines and animal models relevant to DKD for the top ten herbs identified in Chapter 5. The evidence provides biological plausibility and possible explanations for the positive findings shown in clinical trials.

The commonly used herbs are: *huang qi* 黄芪, *dan shen* 丹参, *di huang* 地黄, *shan yao* 山药, *shan zhu yu* 山茱萸, *fu ling* 茯苓, *chuan xiong* 川芎, *da huang* 大黄, *dang gui* 当归 and *ze xie* 泽泻. A review of the common formula is also included, such as *Dong chong xia cao* preparations 冬虫夏草制剂, *Huan shu kui* preparation 黄蜀葵制剂,

Liu wei di huang wan 六味地黄丸, *Jin kui shen qi wan* 金匮肾气丸, and *Bu yang huan wu tang* 补阳还五汤.

Methods

The constituent compounds were identified by searching herbal monographs, high quality reviews of CHM, herbal medicine encyclopedia,[1] materia medica[2] and PubMed. To identify preclinical publications, a literature search of PubMed was undertaken. The search strategy included the terms for each herb and their constituent compounds, *in vitro, in vivo*, DKD, and their synonyms. Studies were screened for relevance in terms of mechanisms of action relevant to DKD. When reviewing and reporting results, scientific methods were considered as well as the impact of the research citations and the journals in which the articles were published. Relevant data were extracted and a summary of the findings are reported here.

Experimental Studies on *huang qi*

Huang qi 黄芪 (*Astragalus membranaceus* var. *mongholicus*) contains several groups of compounds including saponins (astragalosides), flavonoids (quercetin, calycosin), polysaccharides (astraglan), amino acids (palmitic acid) and sterols (β-sitosterol).[1–3] *Huang qi* has been widely researched for its effects on diabetic nephropathy,[4] as well as insulin sensitivity.[5] *Huang qi* has also shown anti-oxidative effects by scavenging free radicals. Free radical damage of the mesangial cells is one of the main pathophysiological mechanisms involved in diabetic nephropathy that causes inflammation around the glomerular blood vessels leading to defective filtration. *Huang qi's* anti-oxidant actions indicate it may have a protective effect against oxidative stress in the early stages of diabetic nephropathy.[3,6] *Huang qi* can also regulate BP, which is a key pathology in people with DKD.[3,7]

The major components of *huang qi*, the astragalosides, have been studied in cell and animal studies. Astragalosides reduced high glucose-induced proliferation of glomerular mesangial cells.[8] The authors concluded that astragalosides may be valuable prophylactics and therapy for DKD because they inhibit cell proliferation and expression of extracellular matrix proteins that are induced by high glucose (a key feature of diabetic nephropathy). In another study, astragaloside IV, was given to rats with streptozotocin (STZ)-induced diabetic nephropathy. Astragaloside IV ameliorated podocyte loss and dysfunction (podocyte destruction is a key feature of diabetic nephropathy caused by oxidative stress leading to proteinuria)[9] and decreased proteinuria, blood glucose levels, and reducing urine albumin.[10,11] Astragaloside I has also been studied in STZ-induced diabetic nephropathy rats.[12] It reduced renal hypertrophy, oxidative stress intensity, blood glucose levels, as well as mesangial hyperplasia and thickness of glomerular base membrane in early stage diabetic nephropathy.

In an *in vivo* study of STZ-induced diabetic rats, the *huang qi* flavonoid quercetin reduced renal dysfunction and oxidative stress via decreasing lipid peroxidation and increasing superoxide dismutase (SOD) and catalase compared to control rats. The authors indicated that quercetin has anti-oxidative mechanisms that may be nephroprotective.[13] Quercetin also reduced high glucose induced mesangial cell proliferation in human mesangial cells.[14] The results indicated that the anti-oxidant effects of quercetin were mediated by nuclear factor-kappaB (NF-κB) signalling. Another major flavonoid, calycosin, also inhibited high glucose-induced rat mesangial cell proliferation.[15]

The anti-oxidant effects of whole extracts of *huang qi* were assessed in STZ-induced diabetic rats. Markers of oxidative stress (malondialdehyde, MDA) and cytokines (tumour necrosis factor alpha; TNF-α) were reduced while activity of antioxidants (SOD) were increased, indicating a potential reduction in kidney damage due to oxidative stress.[16] Taken together, the effects of individual compounds of *huang qi* and whole extracts indicate it has significant potential for preventing, treating and reducing the progression of diabetic nephropathy.

Experimental Studies on *dan shen*

Constituent compounds found in *dan shen* 丹参 (*Salvia miltiorrhiza*) include diterpenoids (tanshinones), phenolic acids (salvianolic acid, ursolic acid), flavonoids and sterols.[1,2] Whole extracts of *dan shen* have been evaluated for their effects in STZ-induced diabetes in rats. Results show that *dan shen* has a number of actions including supressing fibrosis in the renal tubules and glomeruli, and reducing oxidative stress and inflammation by reducing reactive oxygen species (ROS), malondialdehyde and a number of pro-inflammatory factors (TNF-α, interleukin-1beta; IL-1β and interleukin-6; IL-6).[17,18]

The inflammatory response in diabetic nephropathy can be induced and promoted by transforming growth factor beta (TGF-β).[19] A study of the *dan shen* compound, tanshinone A, in glomerular mesangial cells and a rat model of diabetic nephropathy showed suppression of TGF-β, renal hypertrophy and urinary protein excretion.[20] Tanshinone IIA also exhibited reno-protective effects by reducing renal hypertrophy, urinary protein excretion, as well as reducing pro-inflammatory mediators, such as advanced glycation end-products (AGEs), angiotensin II, and TGF-β.[21]

Salvianolic acids isolated from *dan shen* also have anti-oxidant capabilities.[22] In STZ-induced diabetes in mice, salvianolic acid A was associated with reduced macrovascular and renal injury by decreasing oxidative stress, NF-κB expression and modulating nuclear factor E2-related factor 2(Nrf2), a protein that regulates the expression of antioxidants.[23] Other phenolic acids, including ursolic acid and rosmarinic acid, can also prevent biochemical and histo-pathologic changes in the kidneys by reducing inflammation and oxidative stress as well as lowering urine albumin excretion in STZ-induced diabetes in rats.[24,25] Cardiovascular experimental studies also indicate *dan shen* can inhibit angiotensin converting enzyme and lower BP, which may improve renal hypertension in DKD.[26]

Experimental Studies on *di huang*

The constituent compounds in *di huang* 地黄 (*Rehmannia glutinosa*) include glycosides (rehmanniosides, catalpol), adenosine, organic acids, and sterols.[1,2] The glycoside, catalpol, showed anti-diabetic effects in mice by improving insulin resistance and reducing glycated serum protein, insulin, triglycerides, and total cholesterol.[27] This is significant because high levels of circulating insulin increase intra-glomerular pressure causing mesangial expansion and damage to glomerular filtering. The mechanism underlying the hypoglycaemic effects of catalpol have been studied in mice and results showed that it lowered fasting blood glucose by improving mitochondrial function in skeletal muscle cells.[28] Furthermore, catalpol also improved kidney function and reduced pathological changes in STZ-induced diabetes in rats, indicating it may be useful as a preventive against diabetic nephropathy.[29] The reno-protective effects of *di huang* combined with *shan zhu yu* were assessed in a db/db diabetic renal injury mouse model, in which the herb combination decreased serum insulin levels and reduced structural changes in mesangial cells and podocytes in the renal cortex.[30]

The effects of an ethanolic extract of *di huang* were compared to those of metformin in STZ-induced diabetes in rats.[31] Results indicated that metformin was superior at reducing plasma glucose levels but reduction of plasma C-reactive protein, anti-inflammatory activity and antioxidant effects of *di huang* was significant, suggesting reduced diabetes-induced inflammation and oxidative stress. In another study, dried extracts of *di huang* reduced renal histopathological lesions in a high blood glucose rat model. The authors concluded that *di huang* may be useful for inhibiting the progression of diabetic nephropathy.[32]

Experimental Studies on *shan yao*

Saponins (diosgenin, dioscin), phenolic compounds (catecholamine), polysaccharides and sterols are the main compounds in *shan yao* 山药 (*Dioscorea opposite*).[1,2]

Diosgenin isolated from *shan yao* was evaluated in a STZ-induced diabetic rat model for its protective effects on kidney injury.[33] Results showed that diosgenin reduced blood glucose and ameliorated oxidative stress levels by reducing lipid peroxidation and increasing endogenous antioxidant levels. The authors concluded that diosgenin protected the kidneys through antioxidant and anti-inflammatory activities. Allantoin, another compound isolated from *shan yao,* has a similar structure to the anti-diabetic drug metformin. Administration of allantoin to STZ-induced diabetic rats resulted in increased insulin sensitivity by activating imidazoline I-2 receptors in skeletal muscles causing a reduction in blood glucose.[34] This effect appeared to be complementary to that of diosgenin, in that they both improved insulin sensitivity thereby reducing the complications of diabetes.

The saponin dioscin has also shown potent effects by reducing inflammatory kidney injury.[35] *In vivo* injury was induced in rats and mice with an intraperitoneal injection of lipopolysaccharide (LPS) and *in vitro* kidney cells (NRK-52E and HK-2 cells) were challenged with LPS. Dioscin protected against renal damage by inhibiting inflammation, oxidative stress and apoptosis. Whole extracts of *shan yao* have also shown broad antioxidant activities by scavenging ROS.[36] Although the models did not specifically test diabetic nephropathy, dioscin and whole extracts of *shan yao* appeared to exert their therapeutic effects by reducing oxidative stress that may be of significance for inflammatory kidney injury.

Experimental Studies on *shan zhu yu*

The major active compounds in *shan zhu yu* 山茱萸 (*Cornus officinalis*) are isobutanole, glycosides (loganin, cornin, morroniside), tannins (isoterchebin, tellimagrandins) and phenols (ursolic acid, oleanolic acid).[1,2]

Shan zhu yu whole extracts and constituent compounds (including loganin) reduce the expression of collagen IV, fibronectin and IL-6 in glucose-stimulated mesangial cells.[37] Compared to non-treated STZ-induced diabetic rats, the rats given *shan zhu yu* showed reduced urinary albumin, serum creatinine, total cholesterol, and triglycerides as well as reduced oxidative stress by stimulating peroxisome proliferator-activated receptor-gamma (PPARgamma) expression.[38] In another study, an aqueous extract of *shan zhu yu* reduced oxidative stress by restoring enzymatic anti-oxidative defence system and removing reactive molecules in renal tissues in db/db diabetic mice, including lowering the activity of xanthine oxidase, catalase and glutathione S-transferase, enhancing the activity of SOD, and down regulating the mRNA expression of eNOS in kidneys.[39] Morroniside isolated from *shan zhu yu* also inhibited ROS and lipid peroxidation by down-regulating NF-κB, cyclooxygenase-2 (COX-2) and inducible nitric oxide synthase (iNOS).[40] Total triterpene acids from *shan zhu yu* can also reduce oxidative stress and down-regulate TGF-β1.[41] Taken together, *shan zhu yu* appears to have broad effects in reducing oxidative stress.

The glycoside loganin was applied to high glucose stimulated human renal HK-2 cells as well as STZ-induced diabetic rats. *In vitro* connective tissue growth factor (CTGF), a surrogate measure of diabetic nephropathy, was reduced in the HK-2 cells. Renal function also improved in the rat model and logonin reduced serum levels of CTGF indicating it exerts an early renal protective role in diabetic nephropathy.[42] Phenols, including ursolic acid and oleanolic acid, have been extensively researched for their renal protective effects by reducing oxidative and endoplasmic reticulum stress.[24,43,44] In STZ-induced diabetic mice, oleanolic acid inhibited nephropathy by altering spacing between the podocytes, podocyte integrity, and basement membrane thickness, as well as significantly decreasing oxidative stress in the kidneys.[45] In another study, ursolic acid and oleanolic acid were administered to diabetic mice and results showed reduced renal aldose reductase and sorbitol dehydrogenase.[46] Aldose reductase and sorbitol dehydrogenase accumulates in conditions of hyperglycaemia and oxidative stress and advanced kidney disease.

Experimental Studies on *fu ling*

Fu ling 茯苓 (*Poria cocos*) contains triterpenes, polysaccharides, amino acids and organic acids.[1,2] Therapeutic actions of *fu ling* include anti-inflammation, immune-regulation, and anti-cancer.[47] Currently, there are a limited number of experimental studies relevant to the known biochemical pathways involved in diabetic nephropathy.

However *fu ling* and its active constituents, including triterpines (dehydrotumulosic acid, dehydrotrametenolic acid, and pachymic acid), can reduce blood glucose in mice through insulin sensitisation.[48] Dehydrotrametenolic acid can also reduce hyperglycemia in obese hyperglycaemic mice and act as an insulin sensitizer, suggesting that it has promise as a treatment for insulin resistance.[49] *Fu ling* terpenoids also decreased plasma glucose, insulin, triglycerides and inflammatory cytokines, including monocyte chemoattractant protein-1 (MCP-1) and TNF-α. *Fu ling* can also increase anti-inflammatory cytokines, such as adiponectin.[50]

The protective effects of *fu ling* on chronic kidney disease (CKD) induced by adenine were evaluated *in vitro*.[51] *Fu ling* reversed renal injury by regulating biomarkers, including lysoPC(18:0), tetracosahexaenoic acid, lysoPC(18:2), creatinine, lysoPC(16:0) and lysoPE(22:0/0:0) which are commonly identified in CKD, indicating it has anti-fibrotic actions. Ergosterol was also evaluated for its renal protective actions in STZ-induced diabetic mice. Ergosterol significantly reduced blood glucose and biochemical parameters, including uric acid, creatinine, triglycerides, and total cholesterol. In addition to glucose and biochemical parameters, ergosterol also reduced renal pathologic changes in diabetic mice. The results indicated that ergosterol's effects are through suppression of the phosphoinositide 3-kinase (PI3K)/ protein kinase B (Akt)/ nuclear factor-κB (NF-κB) pathways.[52]

Experimental Studies on *chuan xiong*

A wide range of compounds have been identified in *chuan xiong* 川芎 (*Ligusticum chuangxiong*), including phthalides (ligustilide), phenolic compounds (phenylpropanoids), polysaccharides, sterols, and amino acids.[1,2] Phenolic compounds, including caffeic acid and ferulic acid, have been evaluated for their effects on the kidney. A recent review indicated that they can decrease nephrotoxicity and oxidative injury.[53] In STZ-induced diabetic rats, caffeic acid decreased plasma glucose by improving glucose utilisation as well as increasing coronary flow rate.[54] Although kidney tissue was not examined, the results indicate that caffeic acid may also have a positive effect on diabetic nephropathy by reducing the adverse effects of high levels of circulating insulin, including oxidative stress and increased intra-glomerular pressure.

The phenolic compound, ferulic acid, isolated from *chuan xiong* reduced fibrosis in both the hearts and kidneys of hypertensive rats. Systolic blood pressure was significantly reduced, as was inflammatory cell and collagen deposition in the kidneys.[55] Ferulic acid also reduced lipid peroxidation and free radical damage in STZ-induced diabetic rats.[56] Obese diabetic rats given ferulic acid showed similar reduction in oxidative stress as the STZ-induced diabetic rats. Ferulic acid also decreased glomerular basement membrane thickness, glomerular volume, and mesangial matrix expansion, which are the main histopathological changes identified in DKD.[57] Results from these studies indicate that ferulic acid may reduce hypertension and free radical damage associated with diabetes that lead to diabetic nephropathy.

Experimental Studies on *da huang*

Da huang 大黄 (*Rheum palmatum* var. *tanguticum* var. *officinale*) contains anthraquinones, glycosides, tannins, volatile oils and organic acids.[1,2] Active constituents of *da huang,* including anthraquinones (e.g. rhein and emodin) and phenolicacids (e.g. gallic acid and ferulic acid), protect the kidneys by decreasing oxidative stress, inflammation, fibronectin, extracellular matrix accumulation and adverse renal histological changes including fibrosis.[58–60] Rhein has also shown anti-hyperglycaemic effects and lipid lowering activity in obese mice.[58,61] Rhein's influence on cellular hypertrophy, fibronectin synthesis, glucose uptake, and glutamine have been assessed in rat mesangial cells. Rhein increased TGF-βa and p21 expression, in turn decreasing cellular hypertrophy and extracellular matrix synthesis.[62]

When rhein and *dan shen su* 丹参素 from *dan shen* 丹参 were combined, they exerted a synergistic renoprotective effect *in vitro* and *in vivo.*[63] In 5/6 nephrectomised surgery chronic renal injury rats, the administration of rhein and *dan shen su* led to improved renal function and blood supply. Inflammatory cytokines, adhesion molecules, apoptosis and fibrosis were suppressed indicating that combining the two compounds could provide additional renal protection benefits in CKD.

Another anthraquinone compound isolated from *da huang*, emodin, has similar effects to rhein, including anti-diabetic effects in obese mice by lowering blood glucose levels and improving glucose tolerance.[64] In cultured human kidney cells, emodin provided nephroprotection by reducing oxidative stress through scavenging free radicals without decreasing cell viability.[65] In STZ-induced diabetic rats with nephropathy, emodin also inhibited the activation of p38 MAPK pathway and down-regulated the expression of fibronectin thereby ameliorating renal dysfunction.[66]

Whole extracts of *da huang* have been evaluated for their nephroprotective and anti-fibrotic activities. *Da huang* can improve renal function and histopathological abnormalities, including fibrosis and inflammation.[67] Ethanol extracts of *da huang* showed anti-diabetic properties by activating glucose transport in differentiated L6 rat myotubes.[68] Rhaponticin can reduce blood glucose and insulin levels, increase glucose tolerance in KK/Ay type 2 diabetic mice, and reduce triglyceride, cholesterol, low density lipoprotein and non-esterified free fatty acids.[69] In high-fat diet fed and STZ-induced type 2 diabetic rats, gallic acid attenuated insulin resistance through partial agonism of PPARγ and increased glucose uptake via translocating and activating of glucose transporter protein 4(GLUT4) in phosphoinositide 3-kinase/protein kinase B (PI3K/p-Akt) signal pathway.[70] Together, these results indicate that *da huang* and its active constituents may have a significant role to play in insulin regulation and in reducing inflammation and oxidative stress in DKD.

Experimental Studies on *dang gui*

Over 70 compounds have been identified in *dang gui* 当归 (*Angelica sinensis*), including phthalides, volatile oils (carvacrol), fatty acids (oleic acid), amino acids, polysaccharides and sterols (β-sitosterol).[1,2,71]

In STZ-induced diabetic mice, the effects of a *dang gui* polysaccharide was evaluated. After treatment with the polysaccharide, multiple effects were shown, including reduced insulin resistance, serum cholesterol, triglycerides and inflammatory factors IL-6 and TNF-α. The authors concluded that *dang gui* polysaccharide exerted hypoglycaemic and hypolipidemic benefits associated with amelioration of insulin resistance.[72] The volatile oil, carvacrol, extracted from *dang gui* also shows anti-diabetic and anti-hyperglycaemic effects in rats and mice.[73,74] The effects of carvacrol may not be directly related to insulin resistance but rather appears to exert antioxidant properties shown by reduction in alanine aminotransferase, aspartate aminotransferase and lactate dehydrogenase, as well as reduction in serum glucose and cholesterol.

In addition to diabetic effects, *dang gui* appears to exert renal protective effects in studies of diabetic nephropathy. The Japanese variety of *dang gui* (*Angelica acutiloba*) showed anti-diabetic properties and reduced renal injury in STZ-diabetic rats.[75] The effects were shown by a reduction in plasma glucose levels, albumin, and glomerular mesangial matrix expansion, and increase in creatinine clearance. Isoeugenol, isolated from *dang gui* also shows anti-diabetic and renal protective properties due to its antioxidant effects. In STZ-diabetic rats, lipid peroxidation and oxidized glutathione were reduced after isoeugenol treatment thereby effectively reversing diabetic oxidative stress.[76] Succinic acid isolated from *dang gui* also exerted antioxidant effects. STZ-diabetic rats given succinic acid experienced reductions in serum glucose and insulin similar to those achieved with metformin.[77] Succinic acid also reduced serum and tissue lipids and lipid peroxidation, indicating it has additional benefits in terms of anti-peroxidative effects in diabetes.

Experimental Studies on *ze xie*

Ze xie 泽泻 (*Alisma orientalis*) contains triterpenes (alisols), sesquiterpenes (alismol), amino acids and fatty acids.[1,2] The triterpenes, including alisols, have been assessed for their effects on reducing carcinogenesis and hepatotoxicity. However, *ze xie* and its active constituents have a very limited number of studies assessing their benefits in terms of diabetes or diabetic nephropathy.

In vitro, ze xie manifested anti-diabetic properties as evidenced by inhibition of glucose absorption and stimulation of glucose uptake in fibroblasts and adipocytes.[78,79] In STZ-induced diabetic mice, *ze xie* decreased plasma glucose and triglycerides, as well as increased plasma insulin.[80] Unfortunately, the positive effects of *ze xie* have not been followed up and their full effects on diabetes and diabetic nephropathy are yet to be elucidated.

Experimental Studies on Herbal Formulae

Dong chong xia cao preparations 冬虫夏草制剂 (*Cordyceps sinensis*) are single herb formulae commonly used in clinical trials. Constituent compounds include amino acids (aspartic acid, glutamic acid, serine, histidine), fatty acids (oleic acid) and sterols (β-sitosterol).[1,2] Extracts of *dong chong xia cao* have been evaluated for their anti-diabetic effects. In diet-induced and STZ-induced diabetic rats, *dong chong xia cao* exerted a similar effect to metformin in terms of lowering blood glucose (by promoting glucose metabolism), lipids, free radicals (by normalising SOD and glutathione peroxidase levels) and nephropathy.[81] Rats with STZ-induced diabetes showed normalisation of cholesterol, triglycerides, albuminuria and creatinine after *dong chong xia cao.* It also modulated inflammatory factors and oxidative enzymes, which may contribute to improved outcomes in terms of renal protection.[82]

Huang shu kui preparation 黄蜀葵 (*Abelmoschus Manihot* (L.) Medic.) is another single herb formula commonly used in clinical trials. More than 20 constituent compounds have been isolated from *Huang shu kui*, including flavonoids, polysaccharides, tannins and long-chain hydrocarbons. In rats with STZ-induced diabetic nephropathy, total flavone glycosides (TFA) of *Huang shu kui* reduced urine albumin creatinine ratio and 24-h urinary total protein, whilst hyperoside (the main composition of TFA) significantly reduced cultured rat podocyte apoptosis induced by AGEs.[83] In another study, the anti-oxidant and anti-fibrotic effects of whole extraction of *Huang shu kui* were assessed in unilateral nephrectomy and STZ-induced diabetic nephropathy rats. The whole extraction reduced kidney weight, urinary albumin, blood urea nitrogen, and serum uric acid, alleviated renal fibrosis by lowing glomerular cell numbers and glomerular extracellular matrix expansion, and reduced indicators of oxidative stress, including MDA, hydroxy-2'-deoxyguanosine (8-OHdG), total SOD and nicotinamide adenine dinucleotide phosphate (NADPH) oxidase 4 (NOX4). It may exert its anti-fibrotic and anti-oxidant effects via down regulation of the activation of phosphorlyated p38 mitogen-activated protein kinase (p-p38MAPK) and protein kinase B (p-Akt) pathways, as well as the expressions of TGF-β1 and TNF-α.[84] However, neither the whole extraction nor constituent compounds lowered blood glucose level.

Other herbal formulae have been evaluated *in vivo* for their effects on diabetes and diabetic nephropathy. For example, *Liu wei di huang wan* 六味地黄丸, which contains *di huang* 地黄, *shan zhu yu* 山茱萸, *shan yao* 山药, *fu ling* 茯苓, *mu dan pi* 牡丹皮, and *ze xie* 泽泻, has been assessed. Diet and STZ-induced diabetic rats were given *Liu wei di huang wan,* which resulted in reduced fasting blood glucose and fasting insulin levels.[85] These results indicated that *Liu wei di huang wan* can reduce insulin resistance in diabetes. In another study that assessed diabetic nephropathy, a modified *Liu wei di huang wan* (without *shan zhu yu* 山茱萸) reduced serum creatinine and albuminuria and had mild hypoglycaemic effects. *Liu wei di huang wan* also reduced elevated hydroxyproline levels and mesangial expansion, which is one of the main pathological changes of diabetic nephropathy. The study also found that ethanol extracts provided greater effects than water extracts.[86]

The formula, *Jin kui shen qi wan* 金匮肾气丸 also has anti-fibrotic and anti-apoptotic effects. In high-glucose and high-fat diet induced diabetic nephropathy rats, *Jin kui shen qi wan* exerted an anti-fibrotic effect by reducing serum CTGF and TGF-β1. It also increased insulin-like growth factor-1 (IGF-1) and NO excretion in naphridial tissue, reduced plasma endothelin (ET), resulting in reductions in renal vascular pressure and glomerulosclerosis.[87–89] In another study of rats with diet combined with STZ-induced diabetes, *Jin kui shen qi wan* inhibited kidney cells apoptosis by regulating the expression of Bax and Bcl-2 (a pair of genes involved in apoptosis regulation).[90]

The formula, *Bu yang huan wu tang* 补阳还五汤 has been evaluated for anti-oxidant and anti-inflammatory effects on diet and STZ-induced diabetic rats. *Bu yang huan wu tang* lowered blood levels of glucose, nitric oxide (NO) and TNF-α, decreased urinary protein and albumin excretion, and ameliorated insulin resistance.[91] Meanwhile, the expressions of vascular cell adhesion molecule 1 (VCAM-1) and intercellular cell adhesion molecule-1 (ICAM-1) excreted by mesangial cells were down regulated, and renal tubular epithelial cell injury was alleviated.[92]

Other formulae, such as *Dang gui shao yao san* 当归芍药散, *Huang qi dang gui tang* 黄芪当归, 汤, *Wu ling san* 五苓散, *Dang gui bu xue tang* 当归补血汤, etc., have anti-diabetic potential. Their therapeutic effects include antioxidant and anti-inflammatory actions that may reduce the progression of diabetic complications, including diabetic nephropathy.[93–97]

Summary of Pharmacological Actions of the Common Herbs

Experimental research has demonstrated that the frequently used herbs in clinical trials have potent effects on the key mechanisms associated with DKD, including reducing oxidative stress, free radical damage, inflammation, mesangial expansion and fibrosis. The mechanisms of DKD pathogenesis, especially oxidative stress, play a central role in the initiation and progression of diabetic complications.[98] Therefore, the mechanisms of action of the herbal medicines, and their constituent compounds, are central to their role in improving diabetes and diabetic nephropathy.

References

1. Zhou J, Xie G, Yan X. (2011) *Encyclopaedia of Traditional Chinese Medicine: Molecular Structures, Pharmacological Activities, Natural Sources and Applications*. Berlin: Springer.

2. Bensky D, Clavey S, Stoger E. (2004) *Chinese Herbal Medicine: Materia Medica, 3rd ed.* Seattle: Eastland Press.

3. Fu J, Wang Z, Huang L, Zheng S, *et al.* (2014) Review of the botanical characteristics, phytochemistry, and pharmacology of Astragalus membranaceus (Huangqi). *Phytother Res* **28**(9): 1275–1283.

4. Zhang J, Xie X, Li C, Fu P. (2009) Systematic review of the renal protective effect of Astragalus membranaceus (root) on diabetic nephropathy in animal models. *J Ethnopharmacol* **126**: 189–196.

5. Liu H, Guo X. (2007) The effect of APS to f FPG and blood lipids on insulin resistance of rats with type 2D diabetes. *J Mudanjiang Med College* **28**(5): 18–20 [Chinese].

6. Chen C, Zu Y, Fu Y, Luo M, *et al.* (2011) Preparation and antioxidant activity of Radix Astragali residues extracts rich in calycosin and formononetin. *Biocheml Eng J* **56**(1): 84–93.

7. Chen K, Hu J, Xia Q. (2008) Effect of Astragalus membranaceus on hypertension and mechanisms investigation in spontaneously hypertensive rats. *Chin J Lab Diagn* **12**(6): 705–706 [Chinese].

8. Chen X, Wang D, Wei T, He S, *et al.* (2016) Effects of astragalosides from Radix Astragali on high glucose-induced proliferation and extracellular matrix accumulation in glomerular mesangial cells. *Exp Ther Med* **11**: 2561–2566.

9. Li J, Kwak S, Jung D, Kim J, *et al.* (2007) Podocyte biology in diabetic nephropathy. *Kidney Int* **72**: S36–S42.

10. Chen J, Chen Y, Luo Y, Gui D, *et al.* (2014). Astragaloside IV ameliorates diabetic nephropathy involving protection of podocytes in streptozotocin induced diabetic rats. *Eur J Pharmacol* **736**: 86–94.

11. Lu W, Li S, Guo W, Chen L, Li Y. (2015) Effects of Astragaloside IV on diabetic nephropathy in rats. *Genet Mol Res* **14**(2): 5427–5434.

12. Yin X, Zhang Y, Wu H, Zhu X, *et al.* (2004) Protective effects of Astragalus saponin I on early stage of diabetic nephropathy in rats. *J Pharmacol Sci* **95**: 256–266.

13. Anjaneyulu M, Chopra K. (2004) Quercetin, an anti-oxidant bioflavonoid, attenuates diabetic nephropathy in rats. *Clin Exp Pharmacol Physiol* **31**: 244–248.

14. Chen P, Shi Q, Xu X, Wang Y, *et al.* (2012) Quercetin suppresses NF-kappaB and MCP-1 expression in a high glucose-induced human mesangial cell proliferation model. *Int J Mol Med* **30**: 119–125.

15. Tang D, He B, Zheng Z, Wang R, *et al.* (2011) Inhibitory effects of two major isoflavonoids in Radix Astragali on high glucose-induced mesangial

cells proliferation and AGEs-induced endothelial cells apoptosis. *Planta Med* **77**(7): 729–732.

16. Gao Y, Zhang R, Li J, Ren M, *et al.* (2012) Radix Astragali lowers kidney oxidative stress in diabetic rats treated with insulin. *Endocrine* **42**(3): 592–598.

17. Xu L, Shen P, Bi Y, Chen J, *et al.* (2016) Danshen injection ameliorates STZ-induced diabetic nephropathy in association with suppression of oxidative stress, pro-inflammatory factors and fibrosis. *Int Immunopharmacol* **38**: 385–394.

18. Lee S, Kim Y, Lee S, Lee B. (2011). The protective effect of Salvia miltio-rrhiza in an animal model of early experimentally induced diabetic nephropathy. *J Ethnopharmacol* **137**: 1409–1414.

19. Zhu Y, Usui H, Sharma K. (2007) Regulation of Transforming Growth Factor β in Diabetic Nephropathy: Implications for Treatment. *Semin Nephrol* **27**(2): 153–160.

20. Chen G, Zhang X, Li C, Lin Y, *et al.* (2014). Role of the TGFbeta/p65 pathway in tanshinone A-treated HBZY1 cells. *Mol Med Rep* **10**: 2471–2476.

21. Kim S, Jung K, Lee B. (2009) Protective effect of Tanshinone IIA on the early stage of experimental diabetic nephropathy. *Biol Pharm Bull* **32**(2): 220–224.

22. Ho J, Hong C. (2011) Salvianolic acids: Small compounds with multiple mechanisms for cardiovascular protection. *J Biomed Sci* **18**: 30.

23. Wu P, Yan Y, Ma L, Hou B, *et al.* (2016) Effects of the Nrf2 Modulator Salvianolic Acid A Alone or Combined With Metformin on Diabetes-Associated Macrovascular and Renal Injury. *J Biol Chem* **291**(42): 22288–22301.

24. Ling C, Jinping L, Xia L, Renyong Y. (2013) Ursolic Acid provides kidney protection in diabetic rats. *Curr Ther Res Clin Exp* **75**: 59–63.

25. Jiang W, Xu Y, Zhang S, Hou J, Zhu H. (2012) Effect of rosmarinic acid on experimental diabetic nephropathy. *Basic Clin Pharmacol Toxicol* **110**: 390–395.

26. Adams J, Wang R, Yang J, Lien E. (2006) Preclinical and clinical exami-nations of Salvia miltiorrhiza and its tanshinones in ischemic conditions. *Chin Med* **1**: 3.

27. Bao Q, Shen X, Qian L, Gong C, *et al.* (2016) Anti-diabetic activities of catalpol in db/db mice. *Korean J Physiol Pharmacol* **20**(2): 153–160.

28. Li X, Xu Z, Jiang Z, Sun L, *et al.* (2014) Hypoglycaemic effect of catalpol on high-fat diet/streptozotocin-induced diabetic mice by increasing

skeletal muscle mitochondrial biogenesis. *Acta Biochim Biophys Sin (Shanghai)* **46**(9): 738–748.

29. Dong Z, Chen C. (2013) Effect of catalpol on diabetic nephropathy in rats. *Phytomedicine* **20**: 1023–1029.

30. Lv X, Dai G, Lv G, Chen Y, *et al.* (2016) Synergistic interaction of effective parts in Rehmanniae Radix and Cornus officinalis ameliorates renal injury in C57BL/KsJ-db/db diabetic mice: Involvement of suppression of AGEs/RAGE/SphK1 signaling pathway. *J Ethnopharmacol* **185**: 110–119.

31. Waisundara V, Huang M, Hsu A, Huang D, Tan B. (2008) Characterization of the anti-diabetic and antioxidant effects of rehmannia glutinosa in streptozotocin-induced diabetic Wistar rats. *Am J Chin Med* **36**(6): 1083–1104.

32. Yokozawa T, Kim H, Yamabe N. (2004) Amelioration of diabetic nephropathy by dried Rehmanniae Radix (Di Huang) extract. *Am J Chin Med* **32**(6): 829–839.

33. Kanchan D, Somani G, Peshattiwar V, Kaikini A, Sathaye S. (2016) Renoprotective effect of diosgenin in streptozotocin induced diabetic rats. *Pharmacol Rep* **68**: 370–377.

34. Lin K, Yeh L, Chen L, Wen Y, *et al.* (2012) Plasma glucose-lowering action of allantoin is induced by activation of imidazoline I-2 receptors in streptozotocin-induced diabetic rats. *Horm Metab Res* **44**(1): 41–46.

35. Qi M, Yin L, Xu L, Tao X, *et al.* (2016) Dioscin alleviates lipopolysaccharide-induced inflammatory kidney injury via the microRNA let-7i/TLR4/MyD88 signaling pathway. *Pharmacol Res* **111**: 509–522.

36. Liu Y, Li H, Fan Y, Man S, *et al.* (2016) Antioxidant and Antitumor Activities of the Extracts from Chinese Yam (Dioscorea opposite Thunb.) Flesh and Peel and the Effective Compounds. *J Food Sci* **81**(6): H1553–H1564.

37. Ma W, Wang K, Cheng C, Yan G, *et al.* (2014) Bioactive compounds from Cornus officinalis fruits and their effects on diabetic nephropathy. *J Ethnopharmacol* **153**: 840–845.

38. Gao D, Li Q, Gao Z, Wang L. (2012) Antidiabetic effects of Corni Fructus extract in streptozotocin-induced diabetic rats. *Yonsei Med J* **53**(4): 691–700.

39. Kim H, Kim B, Kim Y. (2011) Antioxidative action of corni fructus aqueous extract on kidneys of diabetic mice. *Toxicol Res* **27**(1): 37–41.

40. Park C, Noh J, Tanaka T, Yokozawa T. (2010) Effects of morroniside isolated from Corni Fructus on renal lipids and inflammation in type 2 diabetic mice. *J Pharm Pharmacol* **62**: 374–380.

41. Qi M, Xie G, Chen K, Su Y, *et al.* (2014) Total triterpene acids, isolated from Corni Fructus, ameliorate progression of renal damage in strepto-zotocin-induced diabetic rats. *Chin J Integr Med* **20**(6): 456–461.

42. Jiang W, Zhang S, Hou J, Zhu H.(2012) Effect of loganin on experimental diabetic nephropathy. *Phytomedicine* **19**: 217–222.

43. Lee E, Kim H, Kang J, Lee E, Yadav D, *et al.* (2016) Oleanolic acid and N-acetylcysteine ameliorate diabetic nephropathy through reduction of oxidative stress and endoplasmic reticulum stress in a type 2 diabetic rat model. *Nephrol Dial Transplant* **31**: 391–400.

44. Zhou Y, Li J, Zhang X, Wu Y, *et al.* (2010). Ursolic acid inhibits early lesions of diabetic nephropathy. *Int J Mol Med* **26**(4): 565–570.

45. Dubey V, Patil C, Kamble S, Tidke P, *et al.* (2013) Oleanolic acid prevents progression of streptozotocin induced diabetic nephropathy and protects renal microstructures in Sprague Dawley rats. *J Pharmacol Pharmacother* **4**(1): 47–52.

46. Wang Z, Hsu C, Huang C, Yin M. (2010) Anti-glycative effects of oleanolic acid and ursolic acid in kidney of diabetic mice. *Eur J Pharmacol* **628**: 255–260.

47. Rios J. (2011) Chemical constituents and pharmacological properties of Poria cocos. *Planta medica* **77**(7): 681–691.

48. Li T, Hou C, Chang C, Yang W. (2011) Anti-hyperglycaemic properties of crude extract and triterpenes from Poria cocos. *Evid Based Complement Alternat Med* **2011**: 128402.

49. Sato M, Tai T, Nunoura Y, Yajima Y, *et al.* (2002) Dehydrotrametenolic acid induces preadipocyte differentiation and sensitizes animal models of noninsulin-dependent diabetesmellitus to insulin. *Biol Pharm Bull* **25**(1): 81–86.

50. Kang M, Hirai S, Goto T, Kuroyanagi K, *et al.* (2009) Dehydroabietic acid, a diterpene, improves diabetes and hyperlipidemia in obese diabetic KK-Ay mice. *Biofactors* **35**(5): 442–448.

51. Zhao Y, Feng Y, Bai X, Tan X, *et al.* (2013) Ultra performance liquid chromatography-based metabonomic study of therapeutic effect of the surface layer of Poria cocos on adenine-induced chronic kidney disease provides new insight into anti-fibrosis mechanism. *PLoS One* **8**(3): e59617.

52. Ang L, Yuguang L, Liying W, Shuying Z, *et al.* (2015) Ergosterol Alleviates Kidney Injury in Streptozotocin-Induced Diabetic Mice. *Evid Based Complement Alternat Med* **2015**: 691594.

53. Akyol S, Ugurcu V, Altuntas A, Hasgul R, *et al.* (2014) Caffeic acid phenethyl ester as a protective agent against nephrotoxicity and/or

oxidative kidney damage: A detailed systematic review. *Sci World J* **2014**: 561971.

54. Ho Y, Chen W, Chi T, Chang Chien C, *et al.* (2013) Caffeic acid phenethyl amide improves glucose homeostasis and attenuates the progression of vascular dysfunction in Streptozotocin-induced diabetic rats. *Cardiovasc Diabetol* **12**: 99.

55. Alam M, Sernia C, Brown L. (2013) Ferulic acid improves cardiovascular and kidney structure and function in hypertensive rats. *J Cardiovasc Pharmacol* **61**(3): 240–249.

56. Balasubashini M, Rukkumani R, Viswanathan P, Menon V. (2004) Ferulic acid alleviates lipid peroxidation in diabetic rats. *Phytother Res* **18**: 310–314.

57. Choi R, Kim B, Naowaboot J, Lee M, *et al.* (2011) Effects of ferulic acid on diabetic nephropathy in a rat model of type 2 diabetes. *Exp Mol Med* **43**(12): 676–683.

58. Zeng C, Liu X, Chen G, Wu Q, *et al.* (2014) The molecular mechanism of rhein in diabetic nephropathy. *Evid Based Complement Alternat Med* **2014**: 487097.

59. Ahad A, Ahsan H, Mujeeb M, Siddiqui W. (2015) Gallic acid ameliorates renal functions by inhibiting the activation of p38 MAPK in experimentally induced type 2 diabetic rats and cultured rat proximal tubular epithelial cells. *Chem Biol Interact* **240**: 292–303.

60. Punithavathi V, Prince P, Kumar R, Selvakumari J. (2011) Antihyperglycaemic, antilipid peroxidative and antioxidant effects of gallic acid on streptozotocin induced diabetic Wistar rats. *Eur J Pharmacol* **650**: 465–471.

61. Guo X, Liu Z, Peng A, *et al.* (2002) Rhein retards the progression of type 2 diabetic nephropathy in rats. *Chinese J Nephrol* **18**(4): 280–284 [Chinese].

62. Zheng J, Zhu J, Li L, Liu Z. (2008) Rhein reverses the diabetic phenotype of mesangial cells over-expressing the glucose transporter (GLUT1) by inhibiting the hexosamine pathway. *Br J Pharmacol* **153**: 1456–1464.

63. Guan Y, Wu X, Duan J, Yin Y, *et al.* (2015) Effects and Mechanism of Combination of Rhein and Danshensu in the Treatment of Chronic Kidney Disease. *Am J Chin Med* **43**(7): 1381–1400.

64. Wang Y, Huang S, Feng Y, Ning M, Leng Y. (2012) Emodin, an 11beta-hydroxysteroid dehydrogenase type 1 inhibitor, regulates adipocyte function *in vitro* and exerts anti-diabetic effect in ob/ob mice. *Acta Pharmacol Sin* **33**(9): 1195–1203.

65. Waly M, Ali B, Al-Lawati I, Nemmar A. (2013) Protective effects of emodin against cisplatin-induced oxidative stress in cultured human kidney (HEK 293) cells. *J Appl Toxicol* **33**: 626–630.

66. Wang J, Huang H, Liu P, Tang F, *et al.* (2006) Inhibition of phosphorylation of p38 MAPK involved in the protection of nephropathy by emodin in diabetic rats. *Eur J Pharmacol* **553**(1–3): 297–303.

67. Zhang Z, Wei F, Vaziri N, Cheng X, *et al.* (2015) Metabolomics insights into chronic kidney disease and modulatory effect of rhubarb against tubulointerstitial fibrosis. *Sci Rep* **5**: 14472.

68. Lee M, Sohn C. (2008) Anti-diabetic properties of chrysophanol and its glucoside from rhubarb rhizome. *Biol Pharm Bull* **31**(11): 2154–2157.

69. Chen J, Ma M, Lu Y, Wang L, *et al.* (2009) Rhaponticin from rhubarb rhizomes alleviates liver steatosis and improves blood glucose and lipid profiles in KK/Ay diabetic mice. *Planta Med* **75**(5): 472–477.

70. Gandhi G, Jothi G, Antony P, Balakrishna K, Paulraj M, *et al.* (2014) Gallic acid attenuates high-fat diet fed-streptozotocin-induced insulin resistance via partial agonism of PPARgamma in experimental type 2 diabetic rats and enhances glucose uptake through translocation and activation of GLUT4 in PI3K/p-Akt signaling pathway. *Eur J Pharmacol* **745**: 201–216.

71. Yi L, Liang Y, Wu H, Yuan D. (2009) The analysis of Radix Angelicae Sinensis (Danggui). *J Chromatogr A* **1216**(11): 1991–2001.

72. Wang K, Cao P, Shui W, Yang Q, *et al.* (2015) Angelica sinensis polysaccharide regulates glucose and lipid metabolism disorder in prediabetic and streptozotocin-induced diabetic mice through the elevation of glycogen levels and reduction of inflammatory factors. *Food Funct* **6**: 902–909.

73. Bayramoglu G, Senturk H, Bayramoglu A, Uyanoglu M, *et al.* (2014) Carvacrol partially reverses symptoms of diabetes in STZ-induced diabetic rats. *Cytotechnology* **66**: 251–257.

74. Ezhumalai M, Radhiga T, Pugalendi K. (2014) Antihyperglycaemic effect of carvacrol in combination with rosiglitazone in high-fat diet-induced type 2 diabetic C57BL/6J mice. *Mol Cell Biochem* **385**: 23–31.

75. Liu I, Tzeng T, Liou S, Chang C. (2011) Angelica acutiloba root alleviates advanced glycation end-product-mediated renal injury in streptozotocin-diabetic rats. *J Food Sci* **76**(7): H165–H174.

76. Rauscher F, Sanders R, Watkins J, 3rd. (2001) Effects of isoeugenol on oxidative stress pathways in normal and streptozotocin-induced diabetic rats. *J Biochem Mol Toxicol* **15**(3): 159–164.

77. Saravanan R, Pari L. (2007) Succinic acid monoethyl ester, a novel insulinotropic agent: Effect on lipid composition and lipid peroxidation in streptozotocin-nicotin-amide induced type 2 diabetic rats. *Mol Cell Biochem* **296**: 165–176.

78. Lau C, Chan C, Chan Y, Lau K, *et al.* (2008) *In vitro* antidiabetic activities of five medicinal herbs used in Chinese medicinal formulae. *Phytother Res* **22**: 1384–1388.

79. Li Q, Qu H. (2012) Study on the hypoglycaemic activities and metabolism of alcohol extract of Alismatis Rhizoma. *Fitoterapia* **83**: 1046–1053.

80. Yang X, Huang Z, Cao W, Chen H, *et al.* (2002) Therapeutic and protective effects of water-ethanolic extract from Rhizoma Alismatis on streptozotocin-induced diabetic mice. *Xhongguo Shi Yian Fang Ji Xue Za Zhi* **18**: 336–350 [Chinese].

81. Dong Y, Jing T, Meng Q, Liu C, *et al.* (2014) Studies on the antidiabetic activities of Cordyceps militaris extract in diet-streptozotocin-induced diabetic Sprague-Dawley rats. *Biomed Res Int* **2014**(1): 41–60.

82. Liu C, Song J, Teng M, Zheng X, *et al.* (2016) Antidiabetic and Antinephritic Activities of Aqueous Extract of Cordyceps militaris Fruit Body in Diet-Streptozotocin-Induced Diabetic Sprague Dawley Rats. *Oxid Med Cell Longev* **2016**(3): 1–11.

83. Zhou L, An X, Teng S, Liu J, *et al.* (2012). Pretreatment with the Total Flavone Glycosides of Flos Abelmoschus Manihot and Hyperoside Prevents Glomerular Podocyte Apoptosis in Streptozotocin-induced Diabetic Nephropathy. *J Med Food* **15**: 461–468.

84. Mao Z, Shen S, Wan Y, Sun W, *et al.* (2015) Huangkui Capsule Attenuates Renal Fibrosis in Diabetic Nephropathy Rats through Regulating Oxidative Stress and p38MAPK/Akt Pathways, Compared to α-lipoic acid. *J Ethnopharmacol* **173**: 256–265.

85. Dai B, Wu Q, Zeng C, Cao L, *et al.* (2016) The effect of Liuwei Dihuang decoction on PI3K/Akt signaling pathway in liver of type 2 diabetes mellitus (T2DM) rats with insulin resistance. *J Ethnopharmacol* **192**: 382–389.

86. Liu H, Tang X, Dai D, Dai Y. (2008) Ethanol extracts of Rehmannia complex (*Di Huang*) containing no Corni fructus improve early diabetic nephropathy by combining suppression on the ET-ROS axis with modulate hypoglycaemic effect in rats. *J Ethnopharmaco* **1118**: 466–472.

87. 金智生，李甜，陈雪. (2011) 金匮肾气丸对　2　型糖尿病肾病大鼠 IGF-1 及 ET 的影响. 上海中医药杂志. **45** (11): 76–79.

88. 金智生，陈雪，李甜. (2012) 金匮肾气丸对实验性 2 型糖尿病肾病大鼠血清 TGF- TGF-β1、CTGF 的影响. 中医药学报. **40**(3): 136–139.

89. 金智生，陈雪，李甜. (2012) 金匮肾气丸对实验性 2 型糖尿病肾病大鼠肾组织 NO、NOS 的影响. 中医药学报. **40**(1): 56–59.

90. 姚颖莎，何敏菲，方慧倩，郑燕，张跃明. (2016) 金匮肾气丸对糖尿病大鼠肾脏细胞 Bax、Bcl-2 表达的影响. 浙江临床医学. **18**(4): 595–596.

91. 潘莉，张建新，陈玲燕，马国平，常风云. (2011) 补阳还五汤对 2 型糖尿病大鼠模型血清 TNF-α 及肾脏 VCAM-1 表达的影响. 中国老年学杂志. **31**: 4632–4634.

92. 申晓光. (2009) 补阳还五汤对实验性糖尿病大鼠肾脏 ICAM-1、VCAM-1 表达的影响. 河北医科大学.

93. He K, Li X, Chen X, Ye X, *et al.* (2011) Evaluation of antidiabetic potential of selected traditional Chinese medicines in STZ-induced diabetic mice. *J Ethnopharmacol* **137**: 1135–1142.

94. Liu I, Tzeng T, Liou S, Chang C. (2012) Beneficial effect of traditional Chinese medicinal formula danggui-shaoyao-san on advanced glycation end-product-mediated renal injury in streptozotocin-diabetic rats. *Evid Based Complement Alternat Med* **2012**: 140103.

95. Song J, Meng L, Li S, Qu L, Li X. (2009) A combination of Chinese herbs, Astragalus membranaceus var. mongholicus and Angelica sinensis, improved renal microvascular insufficiency in 5/6 nephrectomized rats. *Vascul Pharmacol* **50**: 185–193.

96. Tzeng T, Liou S, Liu I. (2013) The selected traditional Chinese medicinal formulas for treating diabetic nephropathy: Perspective of modern science. *J Tradit Complement Med* **3**(3): 152–158.

97. Zhang Y, Xie D, Xia B, Zhen R, *et al.* (2006) Suppression of transforming growth factor-beta1 gene expression by Danggui buxue tang, a traditional Chinese herbal preparation, in retarding the progress of renal damage in streptozotocin-induced diabetic rats. *Horm Metab Res* **38**(2): 82–88.

98. Tavafi M. (2013) Diabetic nephropathy and antioxidants. *J Nephropathology* **2**(1): 20–27.

7

Clinical Evidence for Acupuncture and Related Therapies

OVERVIEW

This chapter assesses the clinical evidence of acupuncture and related therapies for diabetic kidney disease. Two randomised controlled trials, one evaluating manual acupuncture and the other point application therapy, showed reductions in urinary albumin excretion. A non-controlled study of moxibustion reported reductions in both urinary albumin excretion and serum creatinine concentration. Overall, there is very little evidence available on acupuncture and related therapies for diabetic kidney disease.

Introduction

Acupuncture is part of a family of techniques which stimulate acupuncture points to correct imbalances of energy and restore health to the body. Methods of stimulating acupuncture points include:

- Manual acupuncture: insertion of acupuncture needles into acupuncture points.
- Moxibustion: burning of a herb (usually *ai ye* 艾叶, *Artemesia vulgaris* L.) close to or on the skin to induce a warming sensation.
- Point application therapy: application of a herbal paste to acupuncture points (also called acupoint sticking therapy or acupoint plaster therapy).

Previous Systematic Reviews

The database search did not find any previous systematic reviews evaluating acupuncture and related therapies for diabetic kidney disease (DKD).

Identification of Clinical Studies

The database search found 33,449 citations. After duplicate removal, 30,499 were screened and 27 articles of acupuncture and related therapies were identified and underwent full-text review. After exclusions, two randomised controlled trials (RCTs) (A1–2) and one non-controlled study were included (A3). There were no non-RCTs (Fig. 7.1). The included studies were conducted in China and published in Chinese journals. Acupuncture techniques used in these trials included manual acupuncture, moxibustion and point application therapy. Each study was summarised separately in the ensuing paragraphs. Acupuncture techniques that are not commonly practiced outside of China are not presented here.

Moxibustion

One RCT (A1) including 60 participants assessed the effect of moxibustion combined with conventional treatments (CTs) and benazepril. Participants' ages ranged from 43 to 70 years. Moxibustion was applied at BL23 *Shenshu* 肾俞 and BL17 *Geshu* 膈俞 for 15 minutes. Treatment was given for six days per week for four weeks. CTs included dietary advice, insulin for blood glucose control and atorvastatin for lipid regulation. Chinese medicine (CM) syndrome was neither used as an inclusion criterion nor as guidance for prescription in the study.

The study used a random number table to generate the allocation sequence. The method for allocation concealment was not described. Blinding of participants and personnel and outcome assessors were at high risk of bias because blinding was not used in the study.

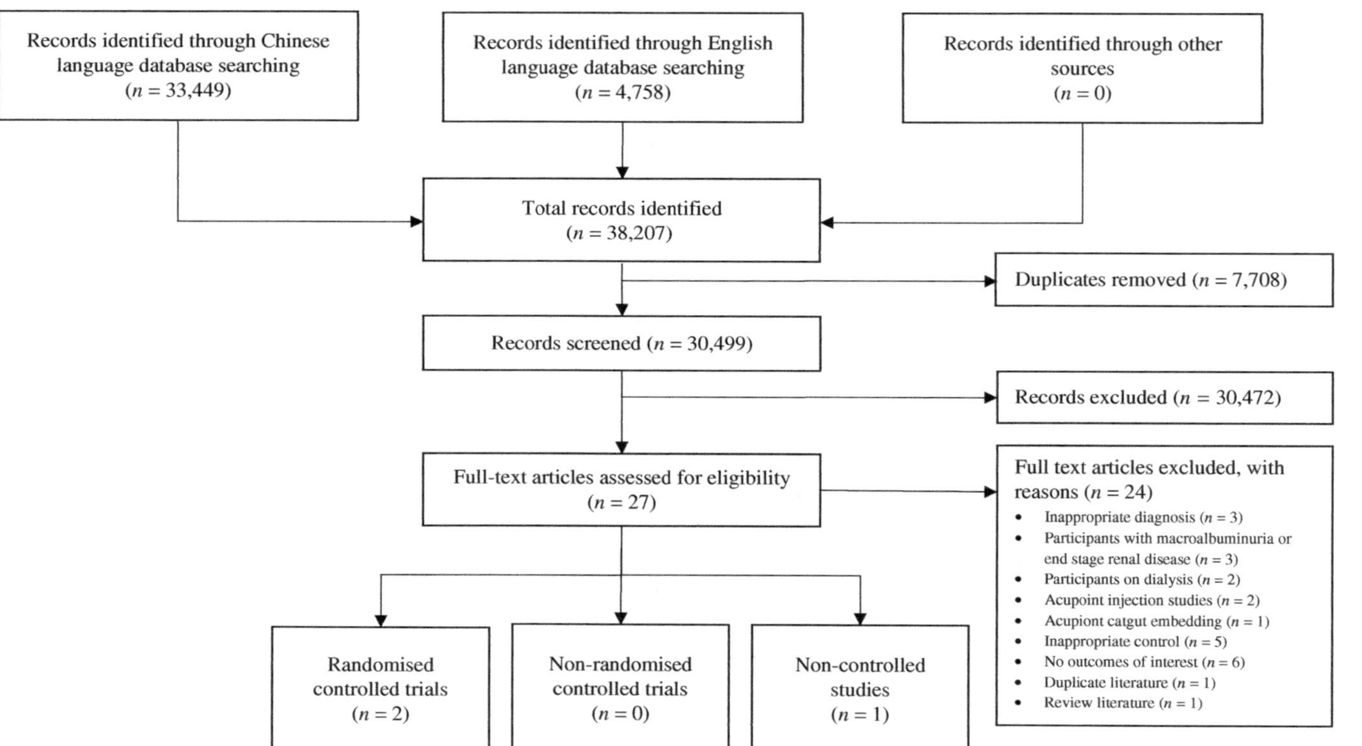

Fig. 7.1. Flow chart of study selection process: acupuncture and related therapies.

Outcome data were complete and there were no missing data or drop-outs. Selective outcome reporting was of unclear risk of bias because the study protocol was not available. Other potential bias risks, including baseline imbalance, were low although commercial funding and potential conflicts of interest were not mentioned. The overall methodological quality of the study was low because there was no blinding of participants and investigators.

Results from the study showed that urinary albumin excretion rate reduced in the moxibustion intervention group compared to CT alone (mean difference (MD) –30.00μg/min [–41.41, –18.59]). The authors did not report if any adverse events occurred during the study.

Acupuncture

One non-controlled case report assessed manual acupuncture in one patient (A3). On the basis of intensive blood glucose control, acupuncture was administered daily for 35 days. CM syndrome diagnosis was not mentioned in this study. The acupuncture points were CV12 *Zhongwan* 中脘, ST36 *Zusanli* 足三里, SP10 *Xuehai* 血海, SP8 *Diji* 地机, ST25 *Tianshu* 天枢, TE6 *Zhigou* 支沟, KI3 *Taixi* 太溪, BL30 *Baihuanshu* 白环俞, BL23 *Shenshu* 肾俞, BL43 *Gaohuang* 膏肓, SP9 *Yinlingquan* 阴陵泉, and CV3 *Zhongji* 中极. The selection of acupoints was based on the treatment methods of reinforcing the Kidney and activating *qi*. At the end of treatment, urinary albumin excretion was reduced from 86.0mg/24h to 35.8mg/24h.

Point Application Therapy

One RCT (A2) compared the effects of point application therapy plus CT to CT alone. The study enrolled 80 participants with an average age of 57 years. Herbal pastes were stuck at the acupoint BL23 *Shenshu* 肾俞 lasting for 30 to 40 minutes. The treatment frequency was twice daily and was continued for 14 days. Herbal paste contained a mixture of *huang qi* 黄芪, *da huang* 大黄, *chuan xiong* 川芎, *dan shen* 丹参, *fu zi* 附子, *chen xiang* 沉香, *xi xin* 细辛, *hong hua*

红花 and vinegar. It should be noted that the use of some herbs, such as *fu zi* and *xi xin*, may be restricted in some countries. Readers are advised to comply with relevant regulations.

The study was at high risk of bias with respect to sequence generation and allocation concealment because the participants were allocated by even and odd numbers of admission. Blinding of participants and personnel and outcome assessors was at high risk of bias because of the nature of the study design. Outcome data were complete and there were no missing data or drop-outs. Selective outcome reporting was at unclear risk of bias because the study protocol was not available. Other potential bias risks, including baseline imbalance, were low although commercial funding and potential conflicts of interest were not mentioned. Overall, the methodological quality of the study was very low.

The study results showed that point application therapy could reduce urinary albumin excretion rate (MD −13.5 µg/min [−20.6, −6.38]) and serum creatinine concentration (−12.4 µmol/L [−20.23, −4.57]). The authors did not report any adverse events.

Summary of Acupuncture and Related Therapies

Acupuncture and related therapies for DKD are not commonly researched in clinical studies. There is limited evidence to support the use of acupuncture therapies for the treatment of DKD. Acupuncture therapies, including manual acupuncture and auricular acupressure, were recommended in CM clinical guidelines (see Chapter 2). However, no studies of auricular acupressure were found, and only a case report showed that manual acupuncture could reduce albuminuria. In addition, the results from the two available RCTs showed that moxibustion and point application therapy may have some positive effects in terms of urinary albumin excretion. BL23 *Shenshu* 肾俞, which was used in both studies, is an acupoint recommended for DKD patients with the syndrome of Kidney deficiency by CM clinical guidelines.[1] However, these two studies were of relatively short duration and low methodological quality. Neither study stated if adverse events occurred. Therefore it is unclear if these therapies are safe and well tolerated by people with DKD. More research is needed to better understand the safety and efficacy of acupuncture treatments for patients with DKD.

References

1. 中华中医药学会糖尿病分会.糖尿病肾脏疾病中医诊疗标准. 世界中西医结合杂志. 2011, **6**(6): 548–552.

References for Included Acupuncture Therapies Clinical Studies

Study Number	Reference
A1	费爱华. (2012) 补肾活血灸法对早期糖尿病肾病疗效和 NO影响. 上海针灸杂志 **31**(12): 891–892.
A2	汪爱民, 尹红, 徐芳. (2013) 中药穴位敷贴透皮给药治疗早期糖尿病肾病的疗效观察. 中国临床护理 **5**(6): 483–485.
A3	ID149 吉学群, 薛莉, 于颂华, 张智龙. (2005) 补肾活血针刺法在糖尿病肾病中的应用. 针灸临床杂志 **21**(1): 43–44.

8

Clinical Evidence for Other Chinese Medicine Therapies

OVERVIEW

Besides Chinese herbal medicine and acupuncture therapies, other types of Chinese medicine therapies have also been used to manage diabetic kidney disease (DKD). This chapter includes clinical evidence of *tai chi* 太极 and Chinese diet therapy for DKD. One randomised controlled trial (RCT) of *tai chi* plus conventional treatment and angiotensin converting enzyme inhibition found significant reductions in both albuminuria and blood pressure. One RCT and a non-randomised controlled trial of Chinese dietary therapy suggested benefits in terms of improving albuminuria, proteinuria, serum creatinine concentration, and blood glucose and lipid control.

Introduction

In addition to Chinese herbal medicine and acupuncture therapies, Chinese medicine (CM) includes a range of therapies to treat disease and maintain health. These include:

- *Tai chi* 太极: A form of mind and body exercise originating from ancient China with a long history based on Chinese Taoist philosophy.
- Chinese diet therapy: The use of foods and herbs to regulate body functions according to individual syndrome differentiation.

Previous Systematic Reviews

The database search did not find any prior systematic reviews evaluating the effectiveness of *tai chi* 太极 and Chinese diet therapy for diabetic kidney disease (DKD).

Identification of Clinical Studies

The database search identified 33,449 citations. After duplicate removal, 30,499 were screened and seven articles of other CM therapies were identified and underwent full-text review. After exclusions, two randomised controlled trials (RCT) (O1, 2) and one non-randomised controlled trial (O3) was included (Fig. 8.1). All three studies were conducted in China and published in Chinese journals. These studies evaluated the effects of *tai chi* 太极 and Chinese diet therapy in addition to CTs. Evidence from each of the studies is presented separately.

Tai chi

One RCT (O1) evaluated the effects of *tai chi* 太极 added to conventional treatments (CTs) with irbesartan. CTs included diet advice, blood glucose and lipid control. The study enrolled 60 participants aged 47 to 75 years old who were randomly allocated to either the *tai chi* or control group. Treatment duration lasted for three months and *tai chi* was performed daily. A total of 24 movements were repeated three to four times in the morning for approximately 1.5 hours.

The study used a random number table to generate the random sequence, but the method for allocation concealment was not described. The study participants and personnel and outcome assessors were not blinded. A full data set was available and there were no missing data drop-outs. Published protocols were not available to judge whether there was selective outcome reporting. Although blinding of personnel is difficult in exercise therapies, including *tai chi*, the methodological quality of the study was downgraded as a result of the lack of blinding.

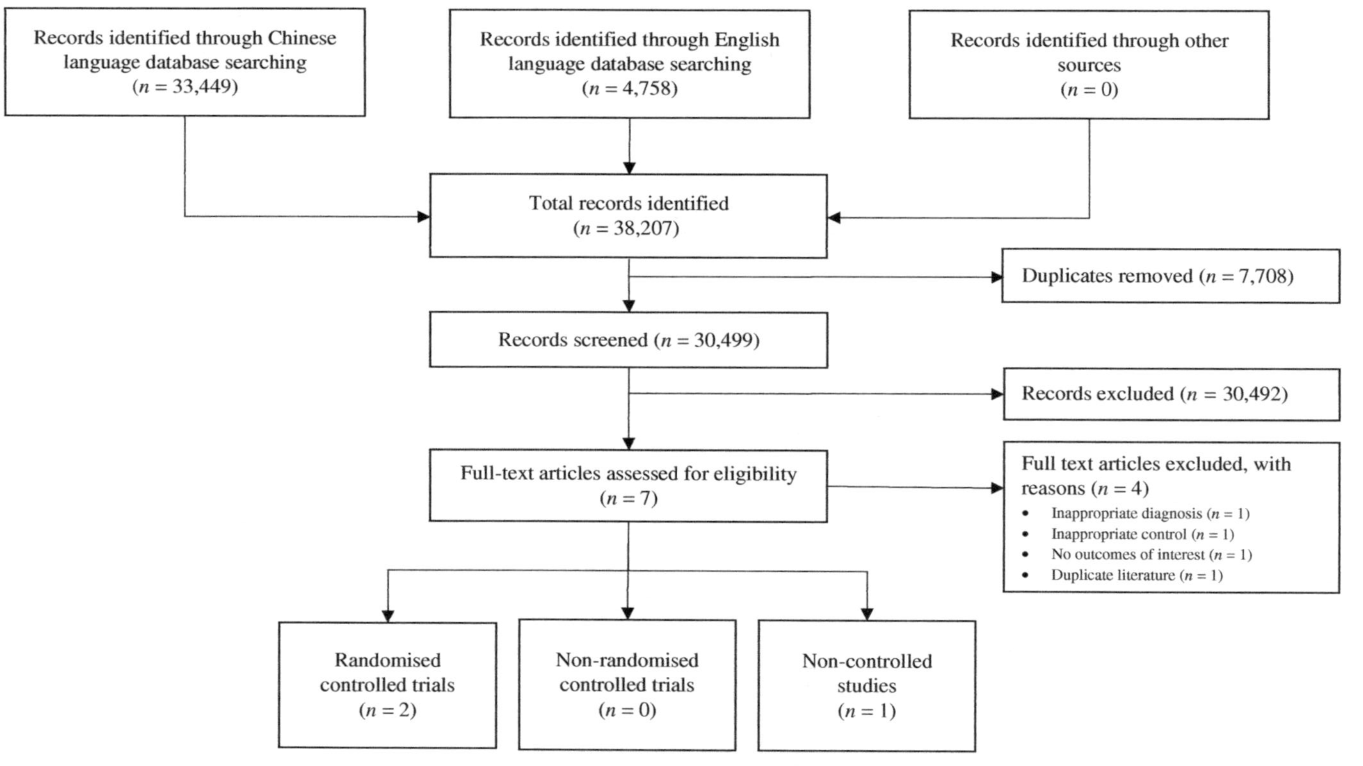

Fig. 8.1. Flow chart of study selection process: other Chinese medicine therapies.

Urinary albumin excretion rate and BP were evaluated after combination treatment and both outcomes improved compared to CT plus irbesartan alone: urinary albumin excretion rate; mean difference (MD) −28.80mg/24h [−39.92, −17.68]; systolic BP MD −18.00mmHg [−20.81, −15.19]; and diastolic BP; MD −6.50mmHg [−8.04, −4.96]. The authors reported that no adverse events occurred during the study period.

Chinese Diet Therapy

One RCT evaluated Chinese diet therapy plus CT compared to CT alone (O2). The CT included diet advice, blood glucose control, BP control and lipid control. The study enrolled 60 DKD patients aged 35 to 70 years with *Spleen* and *Kidney* deficiency. Treatment lasted three months and diet therapy was taken daily. The diet prescription included pork soup for lunch cooked with *shan yao* 山药, *shu di huang* 熟地黄, *ze xie* 泽泻 and *xiao hui xiang* 小茴香.

Although the study was described as "randomised", neither the method for sequence generation nor information on allocation concealment was mentioned. Participants and personnel and outcome assessors were not blinded. The study was assessed as low risk of bias for incomplete outcome data as a full data set of outcomes was available. Selective outcome reporting was at unclear risk of bias because the study protocol was not available. Overall the methodological quality of the study was very low due to the lack of blinding and unclear randomisation sequence generation and allocation concealment.

Urinary albumin excretion rate, serum creatinine concentration and fasting blood glucose level were evaluated. All outcomes were reduced after treatments in both groups, but were reduced to a greater extent in the Chinese diet group compared to the CT group: urinary albumin excretion rate (MD −15.45mg/24h [−22.05, −8.85]), serum creatinine concentration (MD −38.42μmol/L [−42.38, −34.46]), and fasting blood glucose level (MD −1.90mmol/L [−3.15, −0.65]). The authors reported that no adverse events occurred.

One non-randomised controlled study evaluated Chinese diet therapy compared to CT (O3). The CT included diet advice, blood glucose, BP and lipid control. The study enrolled 80 people aged 39 to 68 years with *qi* and *yin* deficiency. Treatment lasted two months and diet therapy was taken daily. The diet prescription included a pork meat pie for lunch cooked with *shan yao* 山药, *shan zha* 山楂, *tian hua fen* 天花粉. The second dish was chicken soup for dinner cooked with *tai zi shen* 太子参, *huang qi* 黃芪, *sheng di huang* 生地黄, and *dan shen* 丹参.

Urinary albumin excretion, urinary protein excretion and fasting blood glucose level were reduced and urine creatinine excretion was increased after treatment in both groups, while total cholesterol and triglycerides were significantly decreased after treatment only in the diet therapy group. Diet therapy showed additional benefits in terms of urinary albumin and protein excretion, fasting blood glucose level, haemoglobin A1c (HbA1c), total cholesterol and triglycerides (Table 8.1). The authors did not report whether any adverse events occurred during the study.

Table 8.1. Effects of the Intervention: Diet Therapy

Outcome (Unit)	Effect Size MD [95% CI]	Included Studies
Urinary albumin excretion rate (μg/min)	−8.85 [−17.59, −0.11]*	O3
Urinary protein excretion (g/24h)	−0.11 [−0.13, −0.09]*	
Urine creatinine (μmol/L)	4.19 [2.33, 6.05]*	
Fasting blood glucose (mmol/L)	−0.78 [−1.57, 0.01]	
HbA1c (%)	−0.26 [−0.48, −0.04]*	
Total cholesterol (mmol/L)	−3.01 [−3.74, −2.28]*	
Total triglycerides (mmol/L)	−1.28 [−1.88, −0.68]*	
HDL-cholesterol (mmol/L)	0.00 [−0.26, 0.26]	

*Statistically significant

Abbreviations: CI, confidence interval; HbA1c, haemoglobin A1c; HDL, high-density lipoprotein; MD, mean difference.

Summary of Other Chinese Medicine

Tai chi 太极 and Chinese diet therapy were evaluated for their effects on DKD. Results indicated that *tai chi* provided a short term benefit in terms of albuminuria reduction and BP control when combined with CTs and irbesartan. Chinese diet therapy may provide benefits in terms of reducing albuminuria, proteinuria and serum creatinine concentration. In addition, diet therapy showed a benefit in regulating blood glucose and lipid levels. The included RCTs showed both *tai chi* and Chinese diet therapy did not produce adverse events. However, due to the small number of studies which were of low or very low methodological quality, the safety and efficacy of these therapies remains unclear and more high quality research with long term follow-up is needed to support the limited positive results.

References for Included Other Chinese Medicine Therapies Clinical Studies

Study Number	Reference
O1	林恒钊. (2012) 厄贝沙坦联合太极拳运动对早期糖尿病肾病的临床疗效观察. 中国民族民间医药 **8**: 108–109.
O2	吴李花, 吴江, 姚景霞. (2014) 中医食疗方在糖尿病 肾病早期的应用效果. 全科护理 **12**(14): 1270–1271.
O3	张穗娥, 董彦敏, 李惠林. (2005) 益气养 阴药膳对早期糖尿病肾病疗效的影响. 广州中医药大学学报 **22**(3): 174–178.

9

Clinical Evidence for Combination Therapies

OVERVIEW

Combination therapies are defined as two or more Chinese medicine interventions administered together, for example, herbal medicine and acupuncture. Two randomised controlled trials were included in this chapter and both studies used Chinese herbal medicine (CHM) combined with acupuncture. The use of combination therapy may improve treatment effectiveness for patients with diabetic kidney disease and microalbuminuria. However, whether the combination is better than CHM alone or acupuncture alone is unknown.

Identification of Clinical Studies

The database search identified 33,449 citations. After duplicate removal, 30,499 were screened and 29 articles of combination therapies were identified and underwent full-text review. After exclusions, two randomised controlled trials (RCT) of Chinese herbal medicine (CHM) combined with acupuncture were included (Fig. 9.1). The combination therapy was compared to different interventions in these two RCTs. Therefore, they were not pooled in meta-analysis.

Chinese Herbal Medicine Combined with Acupuncture

One RCT (C1) compared combination CHM therapy plus CT with angiotensin converting enzyme inhibitors (ACEi) or angiotensin

"

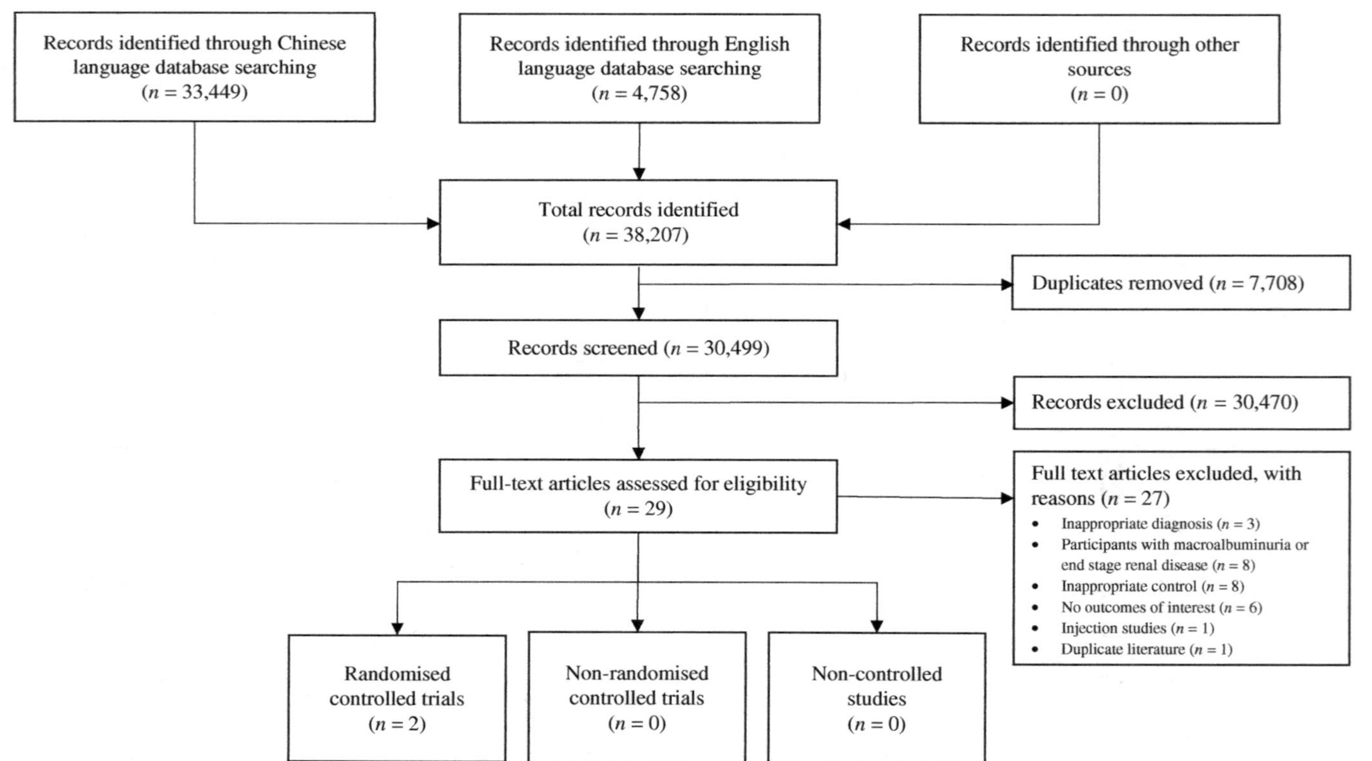

Fig. 9.1. Flow chart of study selection process: combination therapies.

receptor blockers (ARBs) to CT with ACEi/ARB. The other RCT (C2) compared combination therapy to losartan plus CT. Both studies were conducted in China and published in Chinese journals. The studies enrolled 240 participants with microalbuminuria aged from 30 to 76 years. Half of the participants were diagnosed with *qi* and *yin* deficiency plus phlegm and Blood stasis in the meridian (C2). CT included diet and exercise advice, and blood glucose and blood pressure control. Treatments were given daily for six weeks (C1) and two months (C2).

Herb ingredients were unique to each study, except both studies used *bai shao* 白芍, *di long* 地龙, *xuan shen* 玄参 and *shu di huang* 熟地黄. Acupuncture points also differed in each study, but BL23 *Shenshu* 肾俞 and ST36 *Zusanli* 足三里 were used in both studies.

Risk of Bias

The studies used a random number table to generate the allocation sequence, but the method for allocation concealment was not described in either study. Blinding of participants and personnel and outcome assessors was not performed, such that the study was at high risk of bias. There was a low risk for incomplete outcome data because there were no drop outs. Selective outcome reporting was at unclear risk of bias because published protocols were not available. Other potential risks of bias, including baseline imbalance, were low in one study (C1) and high in the other study (C2) because baseline measures were not balanced. Overall the methodological quality of the studies was low due to a lack of blinding.

Outcomes

Combination Therapy Plus CT Plus ACEi/ARB vs. CT Plus ACEi/ARB

Urinary albumin excretion rate (AER) was reported but the data had errors so could not be evaluated (C2). The authors reported positive effects after the combination treatments. Other outcomes were improved including fasting blood glucose level (mean difference, MD −0.60 mmol/L [−1.05, −0.15]); HbA1c (MD −0.20% [−0.36, −0.04]); total cholesterol (MD −1.70 mmol/L [−1.84, −1.56]) and total triglycerides (MD −1.70 mmol/L [−1.79, −1.61]).

Combination Therapy Plus CT vs. ACEi Plus CT

AER was the only outcome reported and was decreased in the combination therapy group compared to the control group (MD −20.93 µg/min [−31.84, −10.02]).

Safety of the Combination Therapies

Both studies did not report whether any adverse events occurred during the study.

Summary of Combination Therapies Evidence

Chinese herbal medicine combined with acupuncture for DKD was evaluated in two RCTs. Combination therapy appeared to reduce blood glucose and lipid levels when added to CT and reduced urinary albumin excretion compared to losartan. Both studies used different herbs and acupuncture points and a firm conclusion about the best combination could not be drawn from the current research. However, some herbs (*bai shao* 白芍, *di long* 地龙, *xuan shen* 玄参 and *shu di huang* 熟地黄) and acupoints (BL23 *Shenshu* 肾俞 and ST36 *Zusanli* 足三里) were used in both studies. *Shu di huang* 熟地黄 was frequently used in CHM studies (refer to Chapter 5) and BL23 *Shenshu* 肾俞, is recommended in clinical guidelines (refer to Chapter 2), and frequently used in acupuncture studies (refer to Chapter 7). The small sample size and low methodological quality of the studies led to uncertainty in the evidence and greatly limited the strength of the conclusions that could be drawn.

It is unclear if other combinations of Chinese medicine therapies would also be effective for DKD. More research is needed to improve the understanding and use of combination therapies for DKD.

References to Included Combination Therapies Clinical Studies

Study Number	Reference
C1	邢晓梅, 王明利, 冯胜奎. (2010) 针药结合治疗早期糖尿病肾病疗效观察. 内蒙古中医药 **16**: 36–37.
C2	张希洲, 占晓芬, 张建新. (2011) 针药结合治疗病 III 期糖尿病肾病 60 例. 四川中医 **29**(5): 116–118.

10

Summary and Conclusions

OVERVIEW

This chapter summarises the main findings of the previous chapters including those dealing with the classical literatures and the clinical trials about Chinese medicine (CM) as treatment for diabetic kidney disease. The current available evidence shows that CM therapies combined with conventional therapy produced promising benefits for the management of diabetic kidney disease. Consistencies and changes of herbal formulae and acupoints from classical to modern use are discussed. The limitations of the available evidence are also discussed, and future directions are identified for further clinical and experimental research.

Introduction

Chinese medicine (CM) therapies have long been used to treat diabetic kidney disease (DKD), and many clinical studies have been conducted. Conventional pharmacotherapies for DKD include glycaemic control, blood pressure (BP) control and lipid management, however, the optimal treatment targets and implementation strategies have not been fully developed and evaluated, and some DKD patients are refractory to current treatments. Therefore, CM treatments may be of value as adjunctive therapy for treating DKD.

This monograph includes a "whole-evidence" synthesis for informing clinical decision-making regarding the role of CM in the management of adults with DKD and microalbuminuria. Clinical guidelines and textbooks have recommended a broad range of CM treatments for DKD, including oral Chinese herbal medicine (CHM), acupuncture, auricular acupressure, herbal retention enema, herbal diet recommendations and lifestyle management (Chapter 2). Review of the classical literature identified a range of herbal medicines which have been used for managing the typical signs and symptoms of DKD (Chapter 3). Hundreds of clinical trials that evaluated the effects of CHM in early DKD were identified. Systematic review and meta-analysis of randomised controlled trials (RCT) demonstrated promising benefits of CHM (Chapter 5). *In vivo* and *in vitro* experimental evidence pertaining to the most frequently used herbs and formulae in RCTs were collected to explore and explain the potential mechanisms of action (Chapter 6). Few clinical trials have been conducted to examine the effects of acupuncture and related therapies for early DKD. Current available evidence suggests that acupuncture and moxibustion therapies may have some benefits (Chapter 7). Evidence regarding other CM therapies for DKD was limited. Only one trial of *tai chi* 太极 and two studies of Chinese diet therapy were found. Further research is needed to assess their benefits (Chapter 8). Research of combinations of CM therapies were lacking as well. Only two clinical trials evaluating CHM with acupuncture were found. Thus, the best combination could not be identified based on current evidence (Chapter 9).

This monograph focused on the evidence for CM therapies in patients with early DKD. Therefore, clinical studies investigating advanced DKD were excluded. Likewise, classical literature records were selected by using the DKD likelihood judgment criteria, such that only historical citations recording the treatments for early DKD were included. However, treatments suggested in CM guidelines and textbooks were recommended for DKD patients (including but not limited to early DKD) with specific CM syndromes rather than with different disease severities.

Chinese Medicine Syndrome Differentiation

Textbooks and CM guidelines recommended that patients be treated according to syndrome differentiation. Seven common CM syndromes were presented with corresponding herbal formula and acupuncture prescriptions, which were proposed to guide clinical practice. However, the majority of CM clinical trials use one formula or a standard acupuncture prescription for all participants. Among these trials, about 40% used CM syndrome as an inclusion criterion or prescribed multiple formulae based on an individual's CM syndrome.

Both in textbooks and guidelines, DKD has been characterised as root deficiency accompanied with excess. Five major deficiency syndromes have been identified, including dual deficiency of *qi* and *yin*, Liver-Kidney *yin* deficiency, dual deficiency of *qi* and Blood, Spleen-Kidney *yang* deficiency and dual deficiency of *yin* and *yang*, and two major excess syndromes are Blood stasis and dampness turbidity (Chapter 2). The deficiency and excess syndromes can be overlapped in individuals and these syndromes are observed in different stages of the disease.

Compared to the syndromes described in Chapter 2, it was found that classification of syndromes in clinical trials (Chapter 5, 7–9) were consistent. For the studies enrolling patients with early DKD that were included in this monograph, *qi* and/or *yin* deficiency were the most common syndromes in clinical trials. Therefore, dual deficiency of *yin* and *yang* and Spleen-Kidney *yang* deficiency, which are common syndromes in advanced stages, were studied to a limited extent or not at all in the included trials. Excess syndrome of Blood stasis was commonly found in clinical trials. Three quarters of CHM trials which assessed CM syndromes reported comorbid Blood stasis syndrome. It should be noted that Blood stasis, which is both the cause and consequence of the pathological process, plays an important role in the disease mechanism of DKD in CM theory.

Commonly used herbs included *huang qi* 黄芪, *shan yao* 山药, *dan shen* 丹参, *di huang* 地黄, *shan zhu yu* 山茱萸, *fu ling* 茯苓, *chuan xiong* 川芎 and *dang gui* 当归, which are categorised as *qi*- and *yin*- tonifying and Blood-activating herbs. This finding suggests that studies which did not report CM syndromes probably enrolled patients with *qi* and/or *yin* deficiency with Blood stasis.

Chinese Herbal Medicine

This section summarises the evidence from Chapters 2, 3 and 5. CHM is the most common form of CM intervention for DKD. The classical literature indicates that the treatment experience of DKD has been passed down from ancient times to the present.

In the classical literature, 88 herbs were identified as treatment for DKD. The high frequency herbs in classical literature, such as *huang lian* 黄连, *ji nei jin* 鸡内金, *tian hua fen* 天花粉 and *zhi mu* 知母, remain widely prescribed to treat diabetes today. The ingredients of *Liu wei di huang wan* 六味地黄丸, including *fu ling* 茯苓, *shu di huang* 熟地黄, *ze xie* 泽泻, *shan yao* 山药, *shan zhu yu* 山茱萸 and *mu dan pi* 牡丹皮, were frequently recorded in classical literature for the treatment of DKD. At present, formulae recommended in serval guidelines, including *Jin kui di huang wan* 金匮肾气丸, *Ji sheng shen qi wan* 济生肾气丸, *Qi ju di huang wan* 杞菊地黄丸, and *Shen qi di huang tang* 参芪地黄汤, were derived from *Liu wei di huang wan* 六味地黄丸. These *di huang* family formulae are commonly used in practice (see Table 5.2).

Apart from traditional and inherited use, there have been developments in modern CHM treatments for DKD. For example, *ren shen* 人参 was one of the most common herbs in ancient records. However, because of its limited yields and high price, *dang shen* 党参 is generally used as a substitute herb in current clinical practice. Formulae like *Sao si tang* 缲丝汤/原蚕茧汤, *Gu ben wan* 固本丸, *Hui xiang san* 茴香散, *Tu si zi san* 菟丝子散, *etc.*, are rarely used in modern CM practice and clinical trials. Researchers have found that the single-herb formula *Sao si tang* (*jian si* 茧丝) exhibited anti-hypoglycaemic and anti-albuminuric effects in pre-clinical studies. This single herb and its active compounds may be candidates for new drug development.

In classical literature, the commonly used herbs were those with Kidney-tonifying and heat-cleaning functions. More recently, ingredients with Blood-activating effects, such as *dan shen* 丹参, *chuan xiong* 川芎, and *dang gui* 当归, have replaced heat-cleaning herbs in modern clinical trials (Table 5.3). This change could be due to a more profound knowledge of disease pathogenesis of DKD with the assistance of modern techniques like microscopy. The typical pathological changes of DKD, such as mesangial matrix expansion, glomerular basement membrane thickening and hemodynamic disturbance, are considered as Blood stasis from a CM perspective, leading to increased utilisation of herbs with Blood-activating features. Accordingly, modern CHM treatment of DKD regularly uses Blood-activating herbs in addition to formulae generated from syndrome differentiation.

Chapter 5 provides a synthesis of the clinical evidence for the effectiveness of CHM in treating early DKD. CHMs were used as an adjunctive treatment to CTs recommended in international guidelines. CTs included diet and exercise advice, blood glucose and blood pressure control, and lipid regulation. There were too few trials using CHM placebo as a comparator to evaluate the absolute effects of integrative therapies (CHMs plus CTs). The difficulty in production of CHM placebo may be the reason why placebo was absent from most of CHM clinical trials.

Most of the treatment and follow up durations were shorter than six months, which was not long enough to adequately observe event end points such as mortality and progression events (progress to end stage renal disease or to advanced stage chronic kidney disease). The majority of clinical trials assessed the effects of CHM using laboratory measurements, including serum creatinine (SCr) concentration, urinary albumin excretion, blood glucose level, BP, *etc.*

In terms of treatment efficacy and safety, evidence from RCTs suggests that:

- Oral CHM added to CTs may reduce SCr concentration in DKD patients with a GFR > 60mL/min, and longer duration may produce greater benefits (low quality evidence), but anti-albuminuric and anti-proteinuric effects were uncertain (very low quality evidence).
- On the basis of CTs, oral CHM plus angiotensin-converting enzyme inhibitors (ACEi) or angiotensin II receptor blockers (ARB)

may further reduce albuminuria and proteinuria compared to ACEi or ARB alone. This beneficial effect was dominated by the subgroup of DKD patients with a GFR ≤ 60 mL/min. It is uncertain whether the risks of mortality and progression were reduced or not by combination treatment (low quality evidence).

- It is uncertain whether oral CHM improves GFR in the short term (very low quality evidence).
- All three treatments, *i.e.*, oral CHM alone, ACEi/ARB alone and CHM plus ACEi/ARB, may reduce BP. The anti-hypertensive effect of ACEi or ARB is superior to that of oral CHM (not graded).
- Compared to hypoglycaemic agents alone, oral CHM plus hypoglycaemic agents made no difference to blood glucose in patients with early DKD (not graded).
- Both oral CHM alone and oral CHM combined with lipid-lowering agents showed a positive effect on regulation of dyslipidaemia (not graded).
- Serious adverse events were not reported in the included studies. However, gastro-intestinal upset and discomfort were observed in some studies. In addition, CHM appeared to reduce the incidence of dry cough caused by ACEi.

Similarities were observed between the commonly reported herbs in clinical trials favouring CHM (Chapter 5, Table 5.17) and the ingredients of formulae recommended in guidelines (Chapter 2). In addition, the ingredients of *Liu wei di huang wan* 六味地黄丸, *huang qi* 黄芪, *chuan xiong* 川芎, *dan shen* 丹参, *dang gui* 当归, which are recommended in guidelines to replenish *qi* and to activate Blood, were frequently used in the RCTs with positive results on kidney function and decreasing albuminuria and proteinuria. The herb *da huang* 大黄 is in the positive herb lists in Chapter 5 as well as the guidelines. For the clinical trials, it was administered orally while in the guideline it was made as decoction and then administered by enema.

Despite evidence generated from clinical trials indicating that a combination of CHM and CTs may be superior to conventional therapies alone, confidence in these results was diminished by the high heterogeneity in meta-analyses and suboptimal methodological quality of included studies. Part of the heterogeneity in the meta-analysis results could be explained by diverse CHM interventions, varied baseline kidney function and albuminuria level, and different treatment durations. Small sample sizes in most of the trials may have contributed to variability as well. Methodology quality was generally considered poor due to lack of blinding, inadequate reporting of the randomisation allocation process, and potential risk of selective outcome reporting in most of the included studies. As for the safety assessment, information about adverse events was not fully provided in all studies. As a result, the quality of evidence from RCTs was downgraded to low or very low in the Grading of Recommendations Assessment, Development and Evaluation (GRADE) assessments.

Chinese Herbal Medicine Formulae in Key Clinical Guidelines and Textbooks, Classical Literature and Clinical Studies

Table 10.1 summarises the CHM formulae described in clinical guidelines and textbooks (Chapter 2), classical literature (Chapter 3), and clinical studies (Chapter 5). Assessment was based on formula name. It is likely that there were formulae with identical or similar herb ingredients but had different names. Assessment of similarity of formulae is complex and was not undertaken, the actual frequency for each listed formula may be higher than reported below.

All typical formulae and products mentioned in Chapter 2 were tested in clinical trials. There were several trials[1-4] evaluating the effects of *Zhen wu tang* 真武汤 and *Fu zi li zhong wan* 附子理中丸, but were not included for further analysis due to use in advanced stages of DKD. Formulae with multiple kinds of evidence are summarised as follow:

- *Jin gui shen qi wan* 金匮肾气丸
  This was the only multi-ingredient formula mentioned in guidelines as well as in classical literature. Evidence from one RCT

Table 10.1. Summary of Chinese Herbal Medicine Formulae

Formula Name	Included in Clinical Guidelines and Textbooks	Included in Classical Literature (No. of Citations)	Included in Clinical Studies (Chapter 5)			Included in Combination Therapies (Chapter 9)
			RCTs (No. of Studies)	CCTs (No. of Studies)	NCS (No. of Studies)	
Bu yang huan wu tang 补阳还五汤	No	0	8	0	0	0
Dong chong xia cao preparations 冬虫夏草制剂	Yes	0	29	0	0	0
Dang gui bu xue tang 当归补血汤	Yes	0	2	0	0	0
Dan zhi jiang tang capsule 丹蛭降糖胶囊	No	0	2	0	0	0
Fu fang xue shuan tong capsule 复方血栓通胶囊	No	0	4	0	0	0
Fu fang dan shen di wan 复方丹参滴丸	No	0	3	0	0	0
Fu zi li zhong wan 附子理中丸	Yes	0	0	0	0	0
Huang kui capsule 黄葵胶囊	Yes	0	4	0	1	0

Jin gui shen qi wan 金匮肾气丸	Yes	4	2	0	0	0
Ji sheng shen qi wan 济生肾气丸	Yes	0	1	0	0	0
Liu wei di huang wan 六味地黄丸	No	4	8	0	0	0
Niao du qing granule 尿毒清颗粒	No	0	4	0	0	0
Nao xin tong capsule 脑心通胶囊	No	0	2	0	0	0
Qi shen yi qi di wan 芪参益气滴丸	No	0	2	0	0	0
Qi zhi jiang tang capsule 芪蛭降糖胶囊	Yes	0	2	0	0	0
Qi ju di huang wan 杞菊地黄丸	Yes	0	0	0	0	0
Qi huang yin (modified) 加味芪黄饮	No	0	2	0	0	0
Qi yao xiao ke capsule 芪药消渴胶囊	No	0	2	0	0	0
Shen qi di huang tang 参芪地黄汤	Yes	0	4	0	0	0

(Continued)

Table 10.1. (*Continued*)

Formula Name	Included in Clinical Guidelines and Textbooks	Included in Classical Literature (No. of Citations)	Included in Clinical Studies (Chapter 5)			Included in Combination Therapies (Chapter 9)
			RCTs (No. of Studies)	CCTs (No. of Studies)	NCS (No. of Studies)	
Shen yan kang fu pian 肾炎康复片	No	0	2	0	0	0
Tong xin luo capsule 通心络胶囊	No	0	5	0	2	0
Xue zhi kang capsule 血脂康胶囊	No	0	6	0	0	0
Yin xing ye preparations 银杏叶制剂	No	0	3	1	0	0
Zhi tang bao shen granule 治糖保肾冲剂	No	0	3	0	0	0
Zhen wu tang 真武汤	Yes	0	0	0	0	0

Abbreviations: CCTs, controlled clinical trials; NCS, non-controlled studies: RCTs, randomised controlled trials.

suggested that *Jin gui shen qi wan* may lower the SCr concentration when used in combination with ACEi plus conventional therapy (low quality evidence). Treatment effect on reducing albuminuria was uncertain (very low quality evidence).

- *Liu wei di huang wan* 六味地黄丸

  This was one of the most common formulae in historical literature, modern clinical trial evidence, and recommended by several guidelines. When compared with ACEi/ARB, pooled estimation of two RCTs favoured *Liu wei di huang wan* in terms of reducing albuminuria (very low quality evidence). When ACEi/ARB plus conventional treatments were applied in both intervention and control groups, urinary albumin and protein excretion may have been further decreased in the group treated with *Liu wei di huang wan* (very low quality evidence). Total cholesterol and low-density lipoprotein level were lower in the CHM group, such that *Liu wei di huang wan* may be beneficial for those with accompanying dyslipidaemia (very low quality evidence).

- *Shen qi di huang tang* 参芪地黄汤

  This formula was recommended in guidelines for *qi* and *yin* deficiency syndrome and used in four RCTs. Evidence generated from an RCT showed that *Shen qi di huang tang* may reduce SCr and albuminuria when used with conventional therapy, regardless of whether it is used in conjunction with ACEi/ARB or not (low quality evidence). It also showed promising results in glycaemic control and dyslipidaemia regulation (not graded).

- *Dang gui bu xue tang* 当归补血汤 and *Ji sheng shen qi wan* 济生肾气丸

  In CM guidelines, *Dang gui bu xue tang* was recommended in combination with *Ji sheng shen qi wan* for the syndrome of dual deficiency of *qi* and Blood. Evidence from an RCT showed that both *Dang gui bu xue tang* combined with benazepril for 6 weeks and *Ji sheng shen qi wan* plus *Fu fang xue shang tong* capsule 复方血栓通胶囊 for 16 weeks may reduce albuminuria (low quality evidence).

- *Bu yang huan wu* tang 补阳还五汤
  Though this formula was not directly mentioned in modern guidelines, its main ingredients were recommended for Blood stasis syndrome. Evidence from RCTs suggested that *Bu yang huan wu tang* may reduce urinary albuminuria excretion regardless of whether it is used with conventional therapy (very low quality evidence) or with ACEi plus conventional therapy (low quality evidence).

- *Qi zhi jiang tang* capsule 芪蛭降糖胶囊
  This multi-ingredient manufactured product was recommended in guidelines for DKD patients with dual deficiency of *qi* and *yin* syndrome with concurrent Blood stasis syndrome. Evidence from one RCT showed that *Qi zhi jiang tang* capsule as an adjunct to CT may reduce albuminuria, and it may be superior to ACEi or ARB (low quality evidence).

- *Dong chong xia cao* preparation 冬虫夏草制剂
  This single ingredient product is a well-established manufactured preparation and its treatment effect has been widely explored in clinical trials. It was recommended in the guidelines as an essence-*qi* enriching agent that is indicated for people with Lung-Kidney *qi* deficiency. Serum creatinine concentration was lower when using *Dong chong xia cao* preparation combined with CT (low quality evidence). When based on ACEi/ARB and CT, *Dong chong xia cao* preparation may not only decrease SCr concentration but also reduce albuminuria excretion (albumin-to-creatinine ratio). These effects only became apparent with a longer treatment duration (more than three months) (low quality evidence).

- *Huang kui* capsule 黄葵胶囊
  This formula contains a single ingredient (*Abelmoschus Manihot* (L.) Medic. Flower) and is indicated for those with dampness-heat syndrome in guidelines. Evidence generated from RCTs showed that the *Huang kui* capsule may reduce albuminuria when added to conventional treatment (low quality evidence). However, this beneficial effect was uncertain when used in combination with ARB plus CT (low quality evidence).

Acupuncture and Related Therapies

This section summarises the evidence from Chapters 2, 3, 7 and 9. In current CM guidelines and textbooks, both manual acupuncture and ear acupressure therapies are recommended for DKD patients. Selection of acupoints is suggested to be according to the CM syndrome of the individual patient. BL23 *Shenshu* 肾俞 (Kidney CO10 肾 in ear) was the only point recommended for all CM syndromes. The points BL20 *Pishu* 脾俞 and SP6 *Sanyinjiao* 三阴交 were recommended for all syndromes except Liver and Kidney *yin* deficiency. These top three most commonly used acupoints are consistent with the core disease mechanism of DKD of deficiency in *qi* and *yin* and disease location in the Kidney and Spleen.

Although a comprehensive search was conducted, only a few classical records and clinical studies of acupuncture and related therapies were found. Two RCTs and one case report used diverse acupuncture therapies, including moxibustion, manual acupuncture and point application therapy. They reported a reduction in urinary albumin excretion in the acupuncture groups, but none of them reported safety outcomes. Furthermore, the poor methodological quality compromised confidence in the results. Consequently, the benefits of acupuncture therapy for patients with DKD remains uncertain.

Acupuncture Therapies in Key Clinical Guidelines and Textbooks, Classical Literature and Clinical Studies

This section summarises and compares the acupuncture therapies and the commonly used acupoints provided in clinical guidelines, textbooks (Chapter 2) and clinical studies (Chapter 7, 9). All acupoints were standardised based on WHO terminology[5] and the frequency of each point was calculated. The traditional points appeared in two or more CM syndromes in Chapter 2 and those overlapping in guidelines and clinical trials (Chapter 2, 7 and 9) are shown in Table 10.2.

Table 10.2.   Summary of Acupuncture and Related Therapies

Acupoints	Included in Clinical Guidelines and Textbooks (Chapter 2)	Included in Classical Literature (Chapter 3) (No. of Citations)	Included in Clinical Studies (Chapter 7) RCTs (No. of Studies)	CCTs (No. of Studies)	NCS* (No. of Studies)	Included in Combination Therapies (Chapter 9)
Acupuncture						
BL23 *Shenshu* 肾俞	Yes	0	0	0	1	2
BL20 *Pishu* 脾俞	Yes	0	0	0	0	1
SP6 *Sanyinjiao* 三阴交	Yes	0	0	0	0	1
GV4 *Mingmen* 命门	Yes	0	0	0	0	1
KI3 *Taixi* 太溪	Yes	0	0	0	1	1
CV4 *Guanyuan* 关元	Yes	0	0	0	0	0
ST36 *Zusanli* 足三里	Yes	0	0	0	1	2
CV3 *Zhongji* 中极	Yes	0	0	0	1	0
BL40 *Weizhong* 委中	Yes	0	0	0	0	1
BL18 *Ganshu* 肝俞	Yes	0	0	0	0	1
BL52 *Zhishi* 志室	Yes	0	0	0	0	1
KI7 *Fuliu* 复溜	Yes	0	0	0	0	1
SP9 *Yinlingquan* 阴陵泉	No	0	0	0	1	1
CV12 *Zhongwan* 中脘	No	0	0	0	1	0
SP8 *Diji* 地机	No	0	0	0	1	1
Moxibustion						
BL23 *Shenshu* 肾俞	No	0	1	0	0	0
BL17 *Geshu* 膈俞	No	0	1	0	0	0
Point Application Therapy						
BL23 *Shenshu* 肾俞	No	0	1	0	0	0
Ear acupuncture						
Kidney CO10 肾	Yes	0	0	0	0	0
Gallbladder CO11 胰胆	Yes	0	0	0	0	0
San Jiao CO17 三焦	Yes	0	0	0	0	0
Endocrine CO18 内分泌	Yes	0	0	0	0	0

*Some studies used more than one intervention, e.g. acupuncture plus moxibustion. These are counted separately in this table.

Abbreviations: CCTs, controlled clinical trials; NCS, non-controlled studies; RCTs, randomised controlled trials.

The commonly used acupoints were located in the meridians of Kidney and Spleen, and were commonly stimulated with supplemental manipulation, which is consistent with the pathogenesis of DKD in CM theory. The acupoint recommended in clinical guidelines for any type of CM syndrome, BL23 *Shenshu* 肾俞, was also used in all clinical studies of acupuncture and related therapies, regardless of operational procedure. However, in current evidence, use of BL23 *Shenshu* 肾俞 was always accompanied with use of other acupoints. Therefore, the precise effect of stimulating BL23 *Shenshu* 肾俞 is uncertain.

Other Chinese Medicine Therapies

This section summarises the evidence from Chapters 2, 3 and 8. In Chapter 2, CM exercises (e.g. *tai chi* 太极 and *ba duan jin* 八段锦) and CM diet therapy are recommended for early stage DKD patients as adjunctive treatments (summarised in Table 10.3). CM diet therapy is suggested according to individual constitution and clinical discomfort. Very few studies evaluated the effects of *tai chi* 太极 and CM diet therapy. Evidence from individual RCTs showed that both therapies, the 24-movement *tai chi* plus irbesartan and CM diet therapy based on CT, may reduce SCr concentration, albuminuria and proteinuria

Table 10.3. Summary of Other Chinese Medicine Therapies

Intervention	Included in Clinical Guidelines and Textbooks (Chapter 2)	Included in Classical Literature (Chapter 3) (No. of Citations)	Included in Clinical Studies (Chapter 8)			Included in Combination Therapies (Chapter 9)
			RCTs (No. of Studies)	CCTs (No. of Studies)	Non-controlled Studies (No. of Studies)	
Tai chi 太极	Yes	0	1	0	0	0
Ba duan jin 八段锦	Yes	0	0	0	0	0
Chinese Diet Therapy	Yes	0	1	0	1	0

Abbreviations: CCTs, controlled clinical trials; RCTs, randomised controlled trials.

without adverse events. However, the evidence for these positive effects was compromised due to limited studies with small sample sizes and suboptimal methodologic quality. Though there were no related records in classical literature, some herbs used in CM diet therapy, such as *xiao hui xiang* 小茴香 and *tian hua fen* 天花粉, were common ingredients in the formulae used to treat DKD in ancient times.

Limitations of Evidence

Despite considerable effort being made to collect and organise data from a wide range of sources, omissions from each of the data sets are possible. In order to present the overview of current CM clinical practice, in Chapter 2, authoritative clinical practice guidelines and textbooks at the time of writing were consulted. Only those CM syndromes and treatments recommended repetitively in different guidelines and textbooks were presented. Therefore, some unusual CM syndromes and potential effective CM treatments which have not been widely acknowledged were not provided in Chapter 2.

In Chapter 3, the sources of classical literature were the CM books included in the *Encyclopaedia of Chinese Medicine (Zhong Hua Yi Dian*, ZHYD, version 5). The ZHYD is considered the largest searchable resource, it does not contain every historical CM text. Thus, missing some CM classical books was unavoidable. There was no specific term in the ancient texts directly referring to DKD as expressed in modern language. To address this, search terms for classical literature were collected from symptoms and signs of DKD and diabetes, and were tested individually. After the expert consensus, three search terms with reasonable specificity were determined, but they may not have been broad enough to capture all possible DKD citations.

The CM books were written by many authors and have been passed down over thousands of years, linguistic changes and errors introduced when copying the manuscripts may have resulted in misinterpretation and/or mistranslation of the intended meaning of some records. Likewise, during the standardised process of herb names, regularisation errors could have been made due to the changes of herbs over time and with location.

Furthermore, as mentioned in Chapter 3, the selection criteria to identify classical citations which were 'possible' or 'likely to be DKD' were established based on signs and symptoms descriptions of the citations. Since the diagnosis of DKD now requires objective laboratory testing, it cannot be confirmed that the citations identified in classical literature were exactly DKD as it is known today. The categories of 'possible DKD' and 'most likely DKD' represent different degrees of confidence of accuracy. Therefore, it cannot be assumed that the herbs and formulae in the 'most likely DKD' group were more effective than those included in the 'possible DKD' group. Similarly, the high frequency herbs and formulae summarised in Chapter 3 can be regarded as potential candidates for further study, but do not necessarily indicate a superior treatment effect.

As for clinical trial evidence, errors of omission or misclassification may have occurred during the process of screening the large number of study records generated by the comprehensive searches. In order to focus on the effects and safety of CM interventions compared to conventional therapies in DKD populations with microalbuminuria, several criteria were applied to exclude studies in which the diagnosis and staging of DKD were unclear. Consequently, some eligible studies may have been excluded due to a lack of detailed information to permit accurate eligibility assessment.

The best available evidence regarding the effects of CM interventions are those generated from RCTs. The reliability of estimated effects increased when the same CM intervention had been tested in multiple RCTs and showed consistent treatment effects. Furthermore, the evidence strengthened if the RCTs were well conducted, rigorous in methodology, sufficient in sample size and representative of the clinical population.

When appropriate, meta-analysis was conducted to provide aggregate data from multiple studies. Of studies included in meta-analysis, variations such as demographic features, condition severity, comorbidity and outcome measurements were considerable. Consequently, substantial statistical heterogeneities were observed in pooled results. Subgroup analyses based on treatment duration, baseline kidney function, CM syndromes and CM formulae were conducted when appropriate and possible to investigate the sources of heterogeneity and provide a more focused evaluation of the treatment effects. The observed heterogeneity could not be completely explained by the above factors, with some factors remaining unknown. Thus, a random effects model was used in all meta-analyses to take into account the clinical heterogeneity and the variation in treatment effects in order to provide conservative estimations of effect sizes.

In the majority of included studies, methodological details of trial design and performance were not adequately reported. Random allocation procedures were not fully described in most of the studies, and neither participants nor investigators were always blinded in the trials. In addition, the quality of reporting of adverse events was unsatisfactory and more detailed information was needed. These deficiencies in methodology and reporting compromised the accuracy of the estimated results, leading to downgrading of the evidence quality.

Due to the large number of eligible studies, it was not feasible to present all details of interventions used in each trial. Thus, the most commonly used CM interventions in the clinical trials, including herbal formulae and their ingredients, acupuncture therapies and acupoints are summarised in the form of frequency tables for each category of evidence. A similar method was used to sum up the high frequency CM interventions applied in the studies included in the meta-analysis, which showed a favourable effect. The downside is that the potential effective CM interventions with low frequency may be submerged under the large volume of data. In order to inform practice and research, the references are provided for people wishing to pursue further research. Also, it should be noted that the most frequently used CM interventions were not the same as the most effective ones.

Participants in all included studies were adults diagnosed with diabetes (either type 1 or type 2) complicated by DKD with microalbuminuria. Consequently, evidence from modern clinical trials cannot be generalised to children, adolescents or those in advanced stages of DKD with macroalbuminuria or uremia. Likewise, since the evidence was based on clinical trials conducted in Asia and the majority of participants were Chinese populations, it is uncertain whether similar treatment effects would be observed in other ethnicities or nationalities. Moreover, the pooled estimations of effect sizes were based on comparisons at the end of treatment. For those meta-analysis showing significant between group differences, it should be carefully examined whether the differences were large enough to be of clinical importance.

The limitations discussed above should be taken into consideration when interpreting the results in the previous chapters.

Implications for Practice

The summary of guidelines and textbooks provides consensus-based expert opinion/guidance for syndrome differentiation and CM treatments for DKD patients. In addition, the study results of classical literature provide background information that may inform clinical practice but should not be used as the basis for clinical decision making.

Even though more than half of the clinical studies did not report CM syndromes, it is likely that *qi* and *yin* deficiency accompanying Blood stasis was the core pathogenesis of DKD based on the most frequently used formulae and herbs.

The available clinical evidence based on laboratory tests of kidney function are very low to low quality. They may indicate that:

- Oral CHMs used as adjunctive therapy for early DKD with micro-albuminuria may reduce albuminuria and SCr concentration, and regulate dyslipidaemia.
- Oral CHMs added to CT may be beneficial for DKD patients with a higher GFR (GFR > 60mL/min), contrary to combination with ACEi or ARB, which shows benefits for DKD patients with a lower GFR (GFR ≤ 60mL/min).

- Longer treatment durations (≥ three months) are required to achieve the clinical benefits of CHMs for DKD patients.
- CHM may reduce the incidence of cough caused by ACEi.
- A small proportion of patients may suffer from gastrointestinal upset when taking CHM. If severe vomiting and/or diarrhoea occur, medicine should be discontinued and the patient should be monitored for potential water and electrolyte disturbances.
- Moxibustion and acupoint application may reduce albuminuria. BL23 *shenshu* 肾俞 should be considered regardless of CM syndrome.
- *Tai chi* 太极 and CM diet therapy may reduce albuminuria.

As the treatment duration and follow up period in most of the included studies was less than six months, the long term benefits of the CM interventions are still unknown. It should be noted that the available evidence was mainly based on populations of Chinese adults. For children, adolescents and other ethnic populations, the differences in physiological and biological characteristics should be taken into consideration in clinical practice.

A known side effect of some toxic herbs is aristolochic acid nephropathy caused by *Aristolochia* L. The herbs reported to be associated with arisotolochic acid nephropathy, e.g. *Aristolochia manshuriensis* Kom (*guan mu tong* 关木通), *Aristolochia fangchi* Y.C. WU *ex* L.D.Chou et S.M.Hwang (*guang fang ji* 广防己) and *Aristolochia debilis* Sieb. et Zucc (*qing mu xiang* 青木香), have been banned in China as well as many countries and areas. Included studies did not use herbs containing aristolochic acid. Of the included studies, however, the insufficient reporting of adverse events and diverse CM interventions led to uncertainty regarding the safety of combination use of CM interventions and conventional pharmacotherapies. Adverse interactions caused by combination of herbs with pharmacotherapy for DKD had not been reported, but attention should be paid and appropriate pharmacovigilance should be applied especially in populations with impaired renal function.

Implications for Research

Despite the fact that a large number of trials evaluating CM interventions for patients with DKD have been conducted, well-designed clinical trials based on a clear hypothesis with long term follow-up are still needed. With due consideration of the limitations of previous studies, recommendations are proposed for further clinical and pre-clinical (experimental) studies.

Clinical Questions

- Perform validation studies to investigate whether CHMs combined with ACEi or ARB reduce albuminuria and the rate of DKD progression in DKD patients with moderate to severe kidney function impairment (SCr >264 μmol/L).
- For different CM interventions, including CHM, acupuncture, moxibustion, *tai chi*, and herbal diet therapy, *etc.*, what are the typical times required for onset of effects and what are the optimal treatment durations?
- Does longer treatment duration always produce better effects for all CM interventions?

Study Design

- Researchers should register their trials with a detailed protocol in a public clinical trial registry before the study starts.
- Methodological experts and statisticians should be involved in trial design at an early stage.
- Strategies to minimise risk of bias should be fully considered when designing the study. Separation of teams to take care of the processes of participant recruitment, random sequence generation and allocation concealment is encouraged. Also, blinding of participants and investigators is desirable whenever possible. The main obstacle to the application of blinding is related to the

nature of CM interventions. For example, decoction is one of the common forms of CHM, which has a specific smell, taste and colour resulting in difficulties manufacturing a matched and identical placebo. These issues can be overcome by processing into the form of capsules, pills and granules thereby facilitating the design of identical control drugs.[6–8] It should be noted that changing from decoctions to powder capsules, pills, or granules may alter the pharmacokinetic and/or pharmacodynamic properties of the ingredients. Data pertaining to the bioequivalence of different forms of CHM are warranted. Similarly, for acupuncture and other manual therapies, the use of sham devices for needle acupuncture, moxibustion and cupping will enhance the feasibility of blinding of participants and personnel in clinical trials.[9–11] If blinding of patients and personnel cannot be achieved, independent outcome assessors and statisticians who are unaware of the treatment allocation can be an alternative. Third party committees (Data Safety Monitoring Boards) should be set up to monitor and collect timely adverse event data and the reasons for dropout cases.

- Clinically important outcomes, such as mortality, progression events and cardiovascular events *etc.*, should be included in study outcomes. Studies with sufficient sample size and a long-term follow-up are required to observe a sufficient number of events.

- Current inconsistency of outcome measurements for albuminuria and proteinuria in clinical trials makes the comparisons of treatment effect across studies more difficult. In recent clinical guidelines, albumin-creatinine ratio was the recommended measurement to monitor the severity of albuminuria for its advantages of convenient sample collection and relatively good accuracy.[12]

- For safety assessment, long term cohort studies or post marketing surveillance studies are often needed in order to obtain reliable data on potential harms.

- Cost-effectiveness analysis should be performed in each clinical trial to provide data for health policy.

Study Reports

Generally, the published CM study reports were too brief to provide sufficient information on methodological design, implementation processes, and the efficacy and safety outcomes. The absence of this information impacts the certainty of the results. Less informative published reports waste research resources. Thus, for future clinical trials, researchers should try to improve the reporting quality of the CM trials. For instance, researchers should adhere to the CARE statement[13] for reporting case reports, the STROBE statement[14] for reporting observational studies, and the CONSORT statement[15] for reporting RCTs. Given the increasing number of clinical studies of CM interventions, the CONSORT extension for acupuncture[16] was published and extension for CHM[17] was updated recently. All of these statements can be obtained from the EQUATOR website (http://www.equator-network.org).

Experimental Studies of Chinese Herbal Medicine

Chapter six briefly summarises the *in vivo* and *in vitro* studies of frequently used herbs for DKD. Most of the previous experimental studies investigated the potential mechanisms of actions/pathways relevant to DKD of a single active compound contained in a herb. However, a single herb contains many compounds, and multiple-ingredient formulae are much more widely used in clinical practice. Therefore, the interactions among multiple compounds, the synergistic or antagonistic effects on the rate of DKD progression would be of considerable interest in future research. In addition, as CHMs are often used as adjunctive therapy in the treatment of DKD, the interactions of herbal compounds and conventional pharmacotherapies are worth further study.

References

1. 申弘道. (2011) 加味真武汤治疗脾肾阳虚型糖尿病肾病 31 例. 河南中医. **31**(9): 970–971.

2. 宋爱军. (2006) 加味真武汤治疗糖尿病肾病少阴证临床与实验研究. 广州中医药大学. 学位论文

3. 胡昌珍. (2012) 真武汤治疗糖尿病肾病 68 例. 中国老年学杂志. **32**(24): 5565–5566.

4. 王向梅. (2007) 真武汤治疗糖尿病肾病疗效观察. 中外健康文摘 · 医药月刊. **11**: 61–63.

5. World Health Organization. (2007) WHO International Standard Terminologies on Traditional Medicine in the Western Pacific Region.

6. Conboy LA, Wasserman RH, Jacobson EE, Davis RB, *et al.* (2006). Investigating placebo effects in irritable bowel syndrome: a novel research design. *Contemp Clin Trials* **27**(2): 123.

7. Li X, Zhang J, Huang J, Ma A, *et al.* (2013) Efficacy and Safety of Qili Qiangxin Capsules for Chronic Heart Failure Study Group. A multi-center, randomized, double-blind, parallel-group, placebo-controlled study of the effects of qili qiangxin capsules in patients with chronic heart failure. *J Am Coll Cardiol* **62**(12): 1065–1072.

8. Tian A, Zhou A, Bi X, Hu S, *et al.* (2017) Efficacy of topical compound Danxiong granules for treatment of dermatologic toxicities induced by targeted anticancer therapy: A randomized, double-blind, placebo-controlled trial. *Evid Based Complement Alternat Med* **3970601**.

9. Tan JY, Suen LK, Wang T, Molassiotis A. (2015). Sham acupressure controls used in randomized controlled trials: A systematic review and critique. *Plos One* **10**(7): e0132989.

10. Zhao BX, Chen HY, Shen XY, Lao L. (2014) Can moxibustion, an ancient treatment modality, be evaluated in a double-blind randomized controlled trial? — A narrative review. *J Integr Med* **12**(3): 131–134.

11. Lee MS, Kim JI, Kong JC, Lee DH, Shin BC. (2010) Developing and validating a sham cupping device. *Acupunct Med* **28**(4): 200–204.

12. National Kidney Foundation. (2007) KDOQI Clinical Practice Guidelines and Clinical Practice Recommendations for Diabetes and Chronic Kidney Disease. *Am J Kidney Dis* **49**: S1–S180 (Suppl 2).

13. Gagnier JJ, Kienle G, Altman DG, Moher D, *et al.* (2013) The CARE Guidelines: Consensus-based Clinical Case Reporting Guideline Development. *Glob Adv Health Med* **2**(5): 38–43.

14. von Elm E, Altman DG, Egger M, Pocock SJ, *et al.* (2014) The Strengthening the Reporting of Observational Studies in Epidemiology (STROBE) Statement: Guidelines for reporting observational studies. *Int J Surg* **12**(12): 1495–1499.

15. Schulz KF, Altman DG, Moher D; CONSORT Group. (2010) CONSORT 2010 statement: Updated guidelines for reporting parallel group randomized trials. *Obstet Gynecol* **115**(5): 1063–1070.
16. MacPherson H, Altman DG, Hammerschlag R, Youping L, *et al.* (2010) Revised Standards for Reporting Interventions in Clinical Trials of Acupuncture (STRICTA): Extending the CONSORT statement. *J Evid Based Med* **3**(3): 140–155.
17. Cheng CW, Wu TX, Shang HC, Li YP, *et al.* (2017) CONSORT Extension for Chinese Herbal Medicine Formulas 2017: Recommendations, Explanation, and Elaboration. *Ann Intern Med* doi: 10.7326/M16–2977.

Glossary

Terms	Acronym	Definition	Reference
95% confidence interval	95% CI	A measure of the uncertainty around the main finding of a statistical analysis. Estimates of unknown quantities, such as the odds ratio comparing an experimental intervention with a control, are usually presented as a point estimate and a 95% confidence interval. This means that if someone were to keep repeating a study in other samples from the same population, 95% of the confidence intervals from those studies would contain the true value of the unknown quantity. Alternatives to 95%, such as 90% and 99% confidence intervals, are sometimes used. Wider intervals indicate lower precision; narrow intervals, greater precision.	http://handbook.cochrane.org/
Angiotensin-converting enzyme inhibitors	ACEi	An oral medicine that lowers blood pressure by inhibiting the body from producing angiotensin II which plays a role in constricting blood vessels.	Nancy K Sweitzer. (2003) What is an angiotensin converting enzyme inhibitor? *Circ* **108**:e16–e18. Levin A, Rocco M. (2007) KDOQI clinical practice guidelines and clinical practice recommendations for diabetes and chronic kidney disease. *Am J Kid Dis* **49**(2):S10–S179.

(Continued)

(*Continued*)

Terms	Acronym	Definition	Reference
Acupressure	—	Application of pressure on acupuncture points	—
Acupuncture	—	The insertion of needles into humans or animals for remedial purposes or its methods	WHO International Standard Terminologies of Traditional Medicine in the Western Pacific Region. World Health Organisation, 2007.
Albumin-creatinine ratio	ACR	The albumin concentration in the urine sample divided by its concentration of creatinine.	
Albumin excretion rate	AER	Albumin excretion rate measures the amount of albumin in the urine.	American Association for Clinical Chemistry (AACC) https://labtestsonline.org
Angiotensin II receptor blockers	ARB	An oral medicine that lowers blood pressure by blocking the action of Angiotensin II.	
Allied and Complementary Medicine Database	AMED	Alternative medicine bibliographic database	https://www.ebscohost.com/academic/AMED-The-Allied-and-Complementary-Medicine-Database
Australian New Zealand Clinical Trial Registry	ANZCTR	Australian clinical trial registry	http://www.anzctr.org.au/
China National Knowledge Infrastructure	CNKI	Chinese language bibliographic database	www.cnki.net
Chinese Biomedical Literature database	CBM	Chinese language bibliographic database	https://cbmwww.imicams.ac.cn
Controlled clinical trials	CCT	An experimental study in which people are allocated to different interventions using methods that are not random.	http://handbook.cochrane.org/
Chinese Clinical Trial Registry	ChiCTR	Chinese clinical trial registry	http://www.chictr.org
Chinese herbal medicine	CHM	Chinese herbal medicine	—
Chinese medicine	CM	—	—

(*Continued*)

(*Continued*)

Terms	Acronym	Definition	Reference
Chongqing VIP Information Company	CQVIP	Chinese language bibliographic database	www.cqvip.com
ClinicalTrials.gov	—	Clinical trial registry	https://clinicaltrials.gov/
Cochrane Central Register of Controlled Trials	CENTRAL	Bibliographic database that provides a highly concentrated source of reports of controlled trials	http://community.cochrane.org/editorial-and-publishing-policy-resource/cochrane-central-register-controlled-trials-central
Combination therapies	—	Two or more Chinese medicines from different therapy groups (e.g. Chinese herbal medicine, acupuncture therapies or other Chinese medicine therapies) administered together.	—
Convention on International Trade in Endangered Species of Wild Fauna and Flora	CITES	—	https://www.cites.org/eng/disc/text.php
Cumulative Index of Nursing and Allied Health Literature	CINAHL	Bibliographic database	https://www.ebscohost.com/nursing/about
Chronic kidney disease	CKD	CKD is defined as abnormalities of kidney structure or function, present for ≥3 months, with implications for health.	Kidney Disease: Improving Global Outcomes (KDIGO) CKD Work Group. KDIGO 2012 Clinical Practice Guideline for the Evaluation and Management of Chronic Kidney Disease. *Kidney Int.*, Suppl. 2013; **3**: 1–150.
Creatinine clearance	CrCl	A creatinine clearance test measures creatinine levels in both a sample of blood and a sample of urine from a 24-hour urine collection. The results are used to calculate the amount of creatinine that has been cleared from the blood and passed into the urine.	American Association for Clinical Chemistry (AACC) https://labtestsonline.org

(*Continued*)

(*Continued*)

Terms	Acronym	Definition	Reference
Conventional treatments	CT	Included various combinations of dietary and lifestyle management, blood glucose control, blood pressure control and/or blood lipid control.	—
Diabetic kidney disease	DKD	Diabetic kidney disease (DKD), previously known as diabetic nephropathy, is a clinical syndrome characterised by persistent albuminuria and progressive loss of kidney function caused by Diabetes Mellitus (DM).	Cheng S, Vijayan A. (2012) *The Washington Manual Nephrology Subspecialty Consult.* 3rd ed. Department of Medicine, Washington University School of Medicine.
Diabetes Mellitus	DM	A condition characterised by hyperglycemia resulting from the body's inability to use blood glucose for energy.	http://www.diabetes.org/ diabetes-basics/ common-terms
Effect size	—	A generic term for the estimate of effect of treatment for a study.	http://handbook.cochrane. org/
EU Clinical Trials Register	EU-CTR	European clinical trial registry	https://www. clinicaltrialsregister.eu
Excerpta Medica dataBASE	Embase	Bibliographic database	http://www.elsevier.com/ solutions/embase
End stage renal disease	ESRD	When loss of kidney function reaches an advanced stage	
Fasting blood glucose	FBG	The amount of glucose in a given amount of blood fasting for at least 8 hours before having a blood glucose test.	http://www.diabetes.org/ diabetes-basics/ common-terms
Glomerular filtration rate	GFR	A measure of the kidneys' ability to filter blood.	National Kidney Foundation. K/DOQI Clinical Practice Guidelines for Chronic Kidney Disease: Evaluation, Classification and Stratification. *Am J Kidney Dis* **39**: S1–S266, 2002 (Suppl 1)

(*Continued*)

(Continued)

Terms	Acronym	Definition	Reference
Grading of Recommendations Assessment, Development and Evaluation	GRADE	Approach used to grade quality of evidence and strength of recommendations.	http://www.gradeworkinggroup.org/
Heterogeneity	—	Used in a general sense to describe the variation in, or diversity of, participants, interventions, and measurement of outcomes across a set of studies, or the variation in internal validity of those studies. Used specifically, as statistical heterogeneity, to describe the degree of variation in the effect estimates from a set of studies. Also used to indicate the presence of variability among studies beyond the amount expected due solely to the play of chance.	http://handbook.cochrane.org/
Homogeneity	—	Used in a general sense to mean that the participants, interventions, and measurement of outcomes are similar across a set of studies. Used specifically to describe the effect estimates from a set of studies where they do not vary more than would be expected by chance.	http://handbook.cochrane.org/
Hemoglobin A1c	HbA1c	A test that measures a person's average blood glucose level over the past 2 to 3 months.	http://www.diabetes.org/diabetes-basics/common-terms
I^2	—	A measure of study heterogeneity, indicates the percentage of variance in a meta-analysis.	http://handbook.cochrane.org/
Integrative medicine	—	Chinese herbal medicine combined with pharmacotherapy or other conventional therapy.	
Kidney Disease Outcomes Quality Initiative guideline	KDOQI	Kidney disease guideline	Levin A, Rocco M. (2007) KDOQI clinical practice guidelines and clinical practice recommendations for diabetes and chronic kidney disease. *Am J Kid Dis* **49**(2): S10–S179.

(Continued)

(Continued)

Terms	Acronym	Definition	Reference
Mean difference	MD	In meta-analysis: A method used to combine measures on continuous scales, where the mean, standard deviation and sample size in each group are known. The weight given to the difference in means from each study (e.g. how much influence each study has on the overall results of the meta-analysis) is determined by the precision of its estimate of effect, mathematically this is equal to the inverse of the variance. This method assumes that all of the trials have measured the outcome on the same scale.	http://handbook.cochrane. org/
Meta-analysis	—	The use of statistical techniques in a systematic review to integrate the results of included studies. Sometimes misused as a synonym for systematic reviews, where the review includes a meta-analysis.	—
Moxibustion	—	A therapeutic procedure involving ignited material (usually moxa) to apply heat to certain points or areas of the body surface for curing disease through regulation of the function of meridians/channels and visceral organs	WHO International Standard Terminologies of Traditional Medicine in the Western Pacific Region. World Health Organisation; 2007.
Non-controlled studies	—	Observations made on individuals, usually receiving the same intervention, before and after an intervention but with no control group.	http://handbook.cochrane. org/
Other Chinese medicine therapies	—	Other Chinese medicine therapies include all traditional therapies except Chinese herbal medicine and acupuncture, such as, *tai chi, qigong, tuina* and cupping.	
Point application therapy	—	Application of a herbal paste to acupuncture points (also called acupoint sticking therapy or acupoint plaster therapy)	

(Continued)

(Continued)

Terms	Acronym	Definition	Reference
Urine protein creatinine ratio	PCR	The protein concentration divided by the creatinine concentration in a spot urine sample.	Ginsberg JM, Chang BS, Matarese RA, Garella S (1983) Use of single voided urine samples to estimate quantitative proteinuria. *N Engl J Med* **309**(25):1543.
PubMed	PubMed	Bibliographic database	http://www.ncbi.nlm.nih. gov/pubmed
Qi gong 气功	—	Physical exercises and breathing techniques	—
Randomised controlled trial	RCT	Clinical trial that uses a random method to allocate participants to treatment and control groups.	—
Risk of bias	—	Assessment of clinical trials to indicate if results may overestimate or underestimate the true effect because of bias in study design or reporting.	http://handbook.cochrane. org/
Risk ratio	RR	The ratio of risks in two groups. In intervention studies, it is the ratio of the risk in the intervention group to the risk in the control group. A risk ratio of one indicates no difference between comparison groups. For undesirable outcomes, a risk ratio that is less than one indicates that the intervention was effective in reducing the risk of that outcome.	http://handbook.cochrane. org/
Serum creatinine concentration	SCr	Creatinine is a waste product of muscle catabolism of the body and protein in the diet. Creatinine is removed from the body by the kidneys. SCr is a measurement of serum level of creatinine.	Stevens LA, Levey AS: (2005) Measurement of kidney function, *Med Clin North Am* **89**: 457–473.
Summary of findings	—	Presentation of results and rating the quality of evidence based on the GRADE approach.	http://www. gradeworkinggroup. org/
Tai chi 推拿	—	Physical exercises and breathing techniques.	—
Urinary protein excretion	UPE	A test that measures the amount of protein being released into the urine.	American Association for Clinical Chemistry (AACC) https:// labtestsonline.org

(Continued)

(*Continued*)

Terms	Acronym	Definition	Reference
Wangfang database	Wanfang	Chinese language bibliographic database	www.wanfangdata.com
World Health Organisation	WHO	WHO is the directing and coordinating authority for health within the United Nations system. It is responsible for providing leadership on global health matters, shaping the health research agenda, setting norms and standards, articulating evidence-based policy options, providing technical support to countries and monitoring and assessing health trends.	http://www.who.int/about/en/
Zhong Hua Yi Dian 中华医典	ZHYD	The Zhong Hua Yi Dian (ZHYD) 'Encyclopaedia of Traditional Chinese Medicine' is a comprehensive series of electronic books on compact disk. The collection was put together by the Hunan electronic and audio-visual publishing house. It is the largest collection of Chinese electronic books and includes the major Chinese ancient works, many of which are from rare manuscripts and are the only existing copies. These books cover the period from ancient times up to the period of the Republic of China (1911–1948).	Hu R, editor. Zhong Hua Yi Dian [Encyclopaedia of Traditional Chinese Medicine]. 4th ed. Chengsha: Hunan Electronic and Audio-Visual Publishing House; 2000.
Zhong Yi Fang Ji Da Ci Dian 中医方剂大辞典	ZYFJDCD	Compendium of Chinese herbal formulae with over 96,592 entries derived from classical Chinese books. The Nanjing Chinese Medicine Institute compiled the ZYFJDCD and first published it in 1993.	Peng H. Zhong Yi Fang Ji Da Ci Dian. Beijing. People's Medical Publishing House; 2005.

Index